METHODS IN MOLECULAR BIOLOGY

Series Editor
John M. Walker
School of Life and Medical Sciences
University of Hertfordshire
Hatfield, Hertfordshire, AL10 9AB, UK

For further volumes
http://www.springer.com/series/7651

The Retinoblastoma Protein

Edited by

Pedro G. Santiago-Cardona

Biochemistry and Cancer Biology Divisions, Basic Science Department, Ponce Health Sciences University, Ponce, Puerto Rico

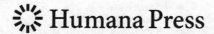 Humana Press

Editor
Pedro G. Santiago-Cardona
Biochemistry and Cancer Biology Divisions
Basic Science Department
Ponce Health Sciences University
Ponce, Puerto Rico

ISSN 1064-3745   ISSN 1940-6029   (electronic)
Methods in Molecular Biology
ISBN 978-1-4939-8522-7   ISBN 978-1-4939-7565-5   (eBook)
https://doi.org/10.1007/978-1-4939-7565-5

Printed on acid-free paper

This Humana Press imprint is published by Springer Nature
The registered company is Springer Science+Business Media, LLC
The registered company address is: 233 Spring Street, New York, NY 10013, U.S.A.

Preface

The retinoblastoma tumor suppressor protein (pRb) not only was the first tumor suppressor to be discovered but also exerts a major tumor suppressive and cell cycle regulatory force in the cell. Most human cancers have an inactivated pRb pathway, thus showing pRb's preeminence as a tumor suppressor, and evidencing the strong anti-oncogenic nature of pRb's function. From early studies of pRb biology emerged the classic and, up until recent years, the predominant paradigm of pRb function, namely pRb as a cell cycle repressor, acting specifically in the G1-S transition checkpoint of the cell cycle. The pRb field has made significant progress in the last decade, and advances have been made in furthering the understanding of the functional and structural aspect of this protein. As a result, a more complex picture is emerging in which pRb acts as a multifunctional protein and master regulator of several aspects of cellular function and homeostasis such as DNA integrity, cell fate choice, lineage commitment, tissue differentiation, apoptosis, senescence and cell adhesion, among others. Consistent with this multiplicity of pRb functions, inactivation of the pRb pathway usually brings about a major disarray in cellular pathways and processes, a scenario that facilitates oncogenic transformation.

Given pRb's predominant role as a regulator of a multitude of cellular functions, and given the pervasive inactivation of pRb in human tumors, assessing the status of pRb and other components of its pathway has become a common practice among cancer researchers studying the cellular and molecular basis of oncogenic transformation. Assessing the status of the pRb pathway components, for example in a tumor biopsy, can dictate treatment options, predict treatment responses, and even potentially inform about survival probabilities.

Together, the chapters in this book have the overarching goal of serving as a laboratory manual that contains protocols and in-depth discussions for commonly used experimental approaches to assess the status and function of components of the pRb pathway, including pRb itself, in cell lines and biological samples. Loss of pRb function in a subset of human cancers such as retinoblastomas, osteosarcomas, and small cell lung carcinomas is primarily due to alterations in the *RB1* gene encoding the pRb protein. Chapter 1 describes a molecular cytogenetics approach to detect deletions of the *RB1* locus, while Chapters 2 and 3 describe methods to assess copy number variations in the *RB1* locus. Tumors harboring a wild type *RB1* gene can nevertheless experience the absence of a functional pRb due to gene silencing by hypermethylation. This topic is addressed in Chapters 4 and 5, which describe methods to assess the methylation status of the *RB1* gene.

From the first five chapters describing approaches to detect genetic and epigenetic mechanisms of pRb inactivation, the book then proceeds to cover mechanisms of pRb inactivation that are of a more biochemical nature. While pRb itself is lost in the subset of human tumors mentioned above, most human tumors show pRb inactivation due to pRb hyperphosphorylation, even in the context of a wild type *RB1* gene. pRb's function is extensively regulated by post-translational modifications, phosphorylation being the predominant one. Therefore, pRb phosphorylation is particularly informative of pRb's functional status. Phosphorylation of pRb within the context of normal cell cycle control results in pRb inactivation, which in turn allows cell proliferation. It is therefore expected that human tumors with wild type *RB1* alleles still show an inactivated pRb due to chronic hyperphosphorylation. Chapter 6 describes an immunoblot protocol to assess pRb phosphorylation in specific residues in protein extracts obtained from either cultured cell lines or tumor tissue samples, while Chapters 7 and 8 describe the immuno-histochemical detection of pRb phosphorylation in human tumor samples. The chronic pRb hyperphosphorylation observed in most human tumors is the consequence of cancer-associated alterations that result either in an overactivation of the Cyclin-dependent kinases (Cdks) that phosphorylate and inactivate pRb or in an inactivation of cellular Cdk inhibitors. In a cancer context, Cdk overactivation can be the result of increased copy numbers of the genetic loci encoding cyclins, which are the regulatory subunits that confer kinase activity to the Cdks. Cyclin D1 amplification is relatively common in human cancers, and therefore assessing Cyclin D1 alterations in tumor samples can be clinically informative. Chapters 9 and 10 describe two methods to assess copy number variations in the Cyclin D1 locus. pRb can still be hyperphos-phorylated in the absence of increased Cdk activity, if important Cdk inhibitors are functionally disrupted. One of such inhibitors is p16, and therefore it is not surprising that p16 inactivation is another noticeable hallmark in human tumors whose assessment in clinical samples can be informative. Chapter 11 describes a protocol to detect p16 silencing by promoter hypermeth-ylation, while Chapter 12 focuses on the immunohistochemical detection of the p16 protein in human tissue samples. In addition to pRb phosphorylation and altered Cyclin D1 and p16 expression, another commonly used surrogate of pRb function is the activity of members of the E2F transcription factor family. pRb's function as a cell cycle repressor requires pRb to antago-nize E2F function, including E2F's DNA binding capacity and transcriptional activation capac-ity. Therefore, pRb and E2F activities are generally considered mutually exclusive mechanistically. Assessment of E2F activity, while not as clinically informative as assessing pRb, p16, and Cyclin D1 status, is nevertheless of high interest and importance for molecular cancer biologists study-ing cellular oncogenesis mechanisms that involve impairment of pRb function. E2F function can be inferred from its capacity to bind E2F-binding sites in several target genes, and this can be assessed by chromatin immunoprecipitation assays, or more directly by measuring its tran-scriptional activation capacity using luciferase reporter gene assays. These two approaches to determine E2F activity are described in Chapters 13 and 14, respectively. Another surrogate of pRb activity is the expression in human tissues of viral oncoproteins that target and inactivate pRb. Some strains of the human papilloma virus (HPV) are oncogenic and therefore detection of the expression of their pRb-targeting oncogenic products can also be informative regarding pRb status. Along these lines, Chapter 15 describes a method to detect HPV E6/E7 mRNA in clinical samples. Finally, Chapter 16 is more geared towards investigators who, rather than assessing pRb status, are interested in manipulating pRb expression to determine the down-stream consequences of such manipulation for cellular function. This chapter describes a CRISPR/Cas-based genomic editing strategy used to abrogate pRb expression.

It is hoped that, taken together, the chapters in this book will allow readers to experi-mentally probe in their laboratories all the many ways in which the function of the pRb tumor suppressor can be altered in a pathological context. The book was designed to cover the mechanisms of pRb inactivation in a manner that is both comprehensive regarding the functionally repressive mechanisms associated with cancer and representative of the experi-mentally relevant tests used in the establishment of cancer diagnosis and prognosis. It is also hoped that the book serves as a guide to assist molecular cancer biologists in their search for understanding of the molecular functions of this preeminent tumor suppressor.

Ponce, Puerto Rico   *Pedro G. Santiago-Cardona*

Contents

Contributors

SUMADI LUKMAN ANWAR • *Department of Surgery, Faculty of Medicine, Universitas Gadjah Mada, Yogyakarta, Indonesia*

MARGIT BALÁZS • *Department of Preventive Medicine, Faculty of Public Health, University of Debrecen, Debrecen, Hungary*

PRIYANKA G. BHOSALE • *Cancer Research Institute, Advanced Centre for Treatment, Research and Education in Cancer (ACTREC), Tata Memorial Centre, Kharghar, Navi Mumbai, India; Homi Bhabha National Institute, Mumbai, India*

MARIA DA GLÓRIA DA C. CARVALHO • *Laboratory of Molecular Pathology, Department of Pathology, Clementino Fraga Filho University Hospital, Federal University of Rio de Janeiro, Rio de Janeiro, Brazil*

MATTHEW J. CECCHINI • *Department of Pathology and Laboratory Medicine, Western University, London, ON, Canada*

JAVED HUSSAIN CHOUDHURY • *Molecular Medicine Laboratory, Department of Biotechnology, Assam University, Silchar, Assam, India*

YASHMIN CHOUDHURY • *Molecular Medicine Laboratory, Department of Biotechnology, Assam University, Silchar, Assam, India*

NEJAT DALAY • *Oncology Institute, Istanbul University, Istanbul, Turkey*

PARTHA PRATIM DAS • *Molecular Medicine Laboratory, Department of Biotechnology, Assam University, Silchar, Assam, India*

RAIMA DAS • *Molecular Medicine Laboratory, Department of Biotechnology, Assam University, Silchar, Assam, India*

FREDERICK A. DICK • *London Regional Cancer Program, Western University, London, ON, Canada; Department of Biochemistry, Western University, London, ON, Canada; Children's Health Research Institute, Western University, London, ON, Canada*

SZILVIA ECSEDI • *MTA-DE Public Health Research Group, University of Debrecen, Debrecen, Hungary*

SANKAR KUMAR GHOSH • *Molecular Medicine Laboratory, Department of Biotechnology, Assam University, Silchar, Assam, India; University of Kalyani, Kalyani, West Bengal, India*

JONATHAN GONZÁLEZ-FLORES • *Biochemistry and Cancer Biology Divisions, Basic Science Department, Ponce Health Sciences University, Ponce, Puerto Rico*

LORRAINE J. GUDAS • *Department of Pharmacology, Weill Medical College of Cornell University, New York, NY, USA*

CHRISTOPHER J. HOWLETT • *Department of Pathology and Laboratory Medicine, Western University, London, ON, Canada*

AINHOA IGLESIAS-ARA • *Department of Genetics, Physical Anthropology and Animal Physiology, University of the Basque Country, UPV/EHU, Bilbao, Spain*

CHARLES A. ISHAK • *London Regional Cancer Program, Western University, London, ON, Canada; Department of Biochemistry, Western University, London, ON, Canada*

CHITRA KANNABIRAN • *Kallam Anji Reddy Molecular Genetics Laboratory, Prof. Brien Holden Eye Research Centre, L.V. Prasad Eye Institute, Hyderabad, India*

GEORGIA KARPATHIOU • *Department of Pathology, University Hospital of St-Etienne, CEDEX2 St-Etienne, France*

VIKTÓRIA KOROKNAI • *MTA-DE Public Health Research Group, University of Debrecen, Debrecen, Hungary*

MANISH KUMAR • *Molecular Medicine Laboratory, Department of Biotechnology, Assam University, Silchar, Assam, India*

SHARBADEB KUNDU • *Molecular Medicine Laboratory, Department of Biotechnology, Assam University, Silchar, Assam, India*

SHAHEEN LASKAR • *Molecular Medicine Laboratory, Department of Biotechnology, Assam University, Silchar, Assam, India*

MIYOUNG LEE • *Aflac Cancer and Blood Disorders Center, Department of Pediatrics, Emory University School of Medicine, Atlanta, GA, USA*

ULRICH LEHMANN • *Institute of Pathology, Medizinische Hochschule Hannover, Hannover, Germany*

THOMAS LIEHR • *Jena University Hospital, Institute of Human Genetics, Friedrich Schiller University, Jena, Germany*

MANOJ B. MAHIMKAR • *Cancer Research Institute, Advanced Centre for Treatment, Research and Education in Cancer (ACTREC), Tata Memorial Centre, Kharghar, Navi Mumbai, India; Homi Bhabha National Institute, Mumbai, India*

THAÍS M. MCCORMICK • *Laboratory of Molecular Pathology, Department of Pathology, Clementino Fraga Filho University Hospital, Federal University of Rio de Janeiro, Rio de Janeiro, Brazil*

ROSY MONDAL • *Institute of Advanced Study in Science and Technology, Guwahati, Assam, India*

ANGEL NÚÑEZ-MARRERO • *Biochemistry and Cancer Biology Divisions, Basic Science Department, Ponce Health Sciences University, Ponce, Puerto Rico*

THOMAS NAERT • *Department of Biomedical Molecular Biology, Ghent University, Ghent, Belgium; Cancer Research Institute Ghent, Ghent, Belgium*

AKISHI OOI • *Department of Molecular and Cellular Pathology, Graduate School of Medical Science, Kanazawa University, Kanazawa, Ishikawa, Japan*

NEREA OSINALDE • *Department of Biochemistry and Molecular Biology, University of the Basque Country, UPV/EHU, Bilbao, Spain*

TAKERU OYAMA • *Department of Molecular and Cellular Pathology, Graduate School of Medical Science, Kanazawa University, Kanazawa, Ishikawa, Japan*

JAILEENE PÉREZ-MORALES • *Biochemistry and Cancer Biology Divisions, Basic Science Department, Ponce Health Sciences University, Ponce, Puerto Rico*

MANISHKUMAR PANDEY • *Cancer Research Institute, Advanced Centre for Treatment, Research and Education in Cancer (ACTREC), Tata Memorial Centre, Kharghar, Navi Mumbai, India*

MICHEL PEOC'H • *Department of Pathology, University Hospital of St-Etienne, CEDEX2 St-Etienne, France*

HAROLD I. SAAVEDRA • *Pharmacology Division, Department of Basic Sciences, Ponce Health Sciences University, Ponce, Puerto Rico*

PEDRO G. SANTIAGO-CARDONA • *Biochemistry and Cancer Biology Divisions, Basic Science Department, Ponce Health Sciences University, Ponce, Puerto Rico*

ISTVÁN SZÁSZ • *MTA-DE Public Health Research Group, University of Debrecen, Debrecen, Hungary*

KRIS VLEMINCKX • *Department of Biomedical Molecular Biology, Ghent University, Ghent, Belgium; Cancer Research Institute Ghent, Ghent, Belgium; Center for Medical Genetics, Ghent University, Ghent, Belgium*

ANA M. ZUBIAGA • *Department of Genetics, Physical Anthropology and Animal Physiology, University of the Basque Country, UPV/EHU, Bilbao, Spain*

Chapter 1

Characterization of *RB1* Deletions in Interphase and Metaphase by Molecular Cytogenetics Exemplified in Chronic Lymphatic Leukemia

Thomas Liehr

Abstract

In chronic lymphatic leukemia (CLL), detection and characterization of prognostic relevant chromosomal alterations is optimally done by interphase-fluorescence in situ hybridization (iFISH). Interphase nuclei derived from blood smears, bone marrow smears or from cultivated and conventionally prepared blood or bone marrow cells can be used. In CLL heterozygous or even homozygous deletion of *RB1* can be found. Interestingly an iFISH diagnostic result with *RB1* deletion as sole aberration is indicative for a favorable course of the disease. Here we describe the best way how to detect *RB1* deletion in CLL.

Key words Tumor cytogenetics, Blood smears, Bone marrow smears, Interphase-fluorescence in situ hybridization (iFISH), Chronic lymphatic leukemia (CLL), RB1 deletion

1 Introduction

As cancer is an age associated disease, in Western countries 1–2% of individuals have to be prepared to obtain the diagnosis "leukemia" during their lifetime [1]. The most frequent leukemia type of advanced age is chronic lymphocytic leukemia (CLL), being a heterogeneous acquired disease. First diagnosis is around 70 years of age; still, as symptoms are mostly unspecific, at time of diagnosis the disease may already be there for several years. A CLL patient may go to see a clinician due to painless enlarged lymph nodes, night sweats, fatigue, fever, weight loss, frequent infections, and/or pain in the upper left portion of the abdomen and enlarged spleen. In ~60% of the cases, CLL progresses very slowly and no treatment is offered to these patients. However, up to 25% of CLL patients progress fast toward acute phase leukemia [2, 3]. To identify high-risk patients and distinguish them from low risk group, molecular cytogenetic diagnostics, like interphase-fluorescence in situ hybridization (iFISH) is routinely performed in CLL [4, 5].

Pedro G. Santiago-Cardona (ed.), *The Retinoblastoma Protein*, Methods in Molecular Biology, vol. 1726,
https://doi.org/10.1007/978-1-4939-7565-5_1, © Springer Science+Business Media, LLC 2018

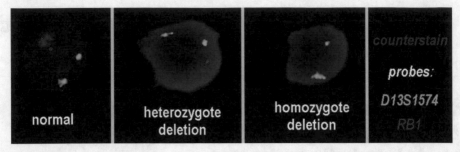

Fig. 1 Three interphase nuclei of one chronic lymphocytic leukemia case with normal signal constitution (left), as well as acquired mosaic heterozygote (middle) and homozyote (right) deletion of the *RB1* locus in the studied cells

Important prognostic markers in CLL comprise mainly deletions in specific chromosomal regions. A favorable course of CLL can be expected if deletions are present exclusively in chromosome 13 including *RB1* gene, while bad prognosis is associated with deletions in chromosome 11 (*ATM* gene) and/or chromosome 17 (*P53* gene). In other words, in case an adverse predicting deletion is found, the CLL patient will receive a different treatment than such patients with favorable genetic markers [4].

iFISH diagnostics can be done on blood or bone-marrow smears or on cultivated and conventionally prepared cells (Fig. 1). Recently we could show that cultured CLL cells are better suited to detect for example *RB1*-deletions than native cells, due to optimal culture conditions for malignant CLL cells using TPA as mitogen [6].

2   Materials

Apart from standard cell biological and molecular cytogenetic equipment, including standard solutions (e.g., ethanol, methanol, formamide, and formaldehyde), no other specialized items are required. The following protocol comprises environmental toxins and teratogens (like formamide and formaldehyde). Please ensure that these substances are collected after use and treated as hazardous waste.

2.1   Smear, Blood, and Bone Marrow Preparation

1. Standard 20× SSC saline sodium citrate (store at RT); set up 2× SSC before use. We purchase the 20× stock in premixed form from Gibco BRL, Cat. No. 15557-036.

2. Carnoy's fixative: methanol–glacial acetic acid 3:1, freshly prepared, at 4 °C.

3. Methanol.

4. Glacial acetic acid.

5. Colcemide.

6. Fetal bovine serum.

7. KCl Hypotonic solution: 0.075 M KCl, freshly prepared.

8. L-Glutamine.

9. Penicillin/streptomycin.

10. TPA = PMA (Phorbol-12-Myristate-13-Acetate).

11. RPMI 1640 medium supplemented with 20% fetal calf serum, 300 μg/ml L-glutamine, 1 U/ml penicillin, 1 μg/ml streptomycin, and 0.4 mg/ml TPA.

12. Standard laboratory slides and 24 × 50 mm coverslips.

13. Standard laboratory incubator with 5% CO_2.

2.2 Fluorescence In Situ Hybridization (FISH)

1. Antifade Vectashield (Cat. No.: H1000, Vector Laboratories/ Biozol; store at +4 °C).

2. DAPI (4,6-diamidino-2-phenylindole, dihydrochloride) stock solution (store at −20 °C).

3. DAPI solution: Dissolve 1.5 μl of a 1 M DAPI stock solution in 1 ml Vectashield antifade (store at +4 °C; can be used at least for 3 months).

4. Denaturation buffer: 70% (v/v) formamide, 20% (v/v) filtered double distilled water, 10% (v/v) 20× SSC; make fresh as required.

5. Ethanol 100, 90 and 70% (store at room temperature).

6. Formamide (aliquot and store at −20 °C).

7. PBS 1× (phosphate buffered saline, store at room temperature). We purchase this in premixed form (Biochrom Cat. No. L825).

8. Rubber cement: Fixogum™.

9. Standard 20× SSC saline sodium citrate (store at RT); set up 2× SSC before use. We purchase the 20× stock in premixed form from Gibco BRL, Cat. No. 15557-036.

10. Zyto*Light*® SPEC RB1/13q12 Dual Color Probe (Cat. No. Z-2165-50, ZytoVision).

11. Standard laboratory warming plate.

12. Coplin jars.

13. Humid chamber for incubating slides.

3 Methods

3.1 Smear Preparation

1. Drop 100–200 μl of the blood or bone marrow onto one end of a dry and clean slide.

2. Spread the fluid along the slide using the small edge of a 24 × 50 mm coverslip. The edge of the coverslip is moved

slowly only one time over the slide; the coverslip must not touch the slide surface (*see* **Note 1**).

3. Let the fluid dry out at room temperature (RT) for approx. 12 h, before performing the slide pretreatment (*see* **Note 2**).

4. Rinse in 2× SSC for 5 min and allow to air-dry.

3.2 Blood and Bone Marrow Preparation

In addition to preparing smears from blood, bone marrow or effusions as described above, this material may also be prepared as described below; this leads to interphase cell suspension in methanol–glacial acetic acid (3:1) which can be stored for years at −20 °C.

1. Add 1 ml of heparinized blood or bone marrow to 9 ml of RPMI 1640 cell culture medium (*see* **Note 3**), mix carefully, and incubate for 96 h at 37 °C in 5% CO_2. **Steps 1** and **2** must be performed under sterile conditions (*see* **Note 4**).

2. 95.5 h later add 1 μg of colcemide to the culture, mix gently, and incubate again for 30 min at 37 °C in 5% CO_2.

3. Working under nonsterile conditions, transfer the fluid into a 15 ml tube.

4. Centrifuge the solution at RT for 8 min at 900 × *g*, and discard the supernatant (*see* **Note 5**).

5. Resuspend the pellet in 10 ml 0.075 M KCl (37 °C) and incubate at 37 °C for 20 min (this is the hypotonic treatment step).

6. Add slowly 0.6 ml of Carnoy's fixative (4 °C) and mix the solution carefully.

7. Repeat **step 4**.

8. Resuspend the pellet in 10 ml of fixative (4 °C) and incubate at 4 °C for 20 min.

9. Repeat **step 4**.

10. Resuspend the pellet in 5 ml of fixative (4 °C) and repeat **step 4**.

11. Repeat **step 10** twice.

12. Resuspend the pellet finally in 0.3–1 ml of fixative (depending on the density of the suspension).

13. Place 1–2 drops of the suspension onto a clean and humid slide using a glass pipette and let the slide dry at RT.

14. After incubation overnight at RT, the slides can be rinsed with 2× SSC.

3.3 Fluorescence In Situ Hybridization (FISH)

FISH is done here using a commercial probe specific for *RB1*. Thus, here we provide a general FISH protocol.

1. FISH probes (here Zyto*Light*® SPEC RB1/13q12 Dual Color Probe (Cat. No. Z-2165-50, ZytoVision) need to be treated according to the manufacturer's instructions; most often this

just means to dilute a certain amount of labeled probe with a hybridization solution provided by the manufacturer.

2. Denature the corresponding solution in a 0.5 or 1.5 ml reaction cup at 75 °C for 5 min (*see* **Note 6**).

3. Store probe on ice until applied to the denatured slide in **step 9** (*see* **Note 7**).

4. Dehydrate slide(s) with interphase nuclei in an ethanol series (70%, 90%, and 100%, 3 min each) and air-dry.

5. Add 100 μl of denaturation buffer to the slide(s) and cover with 24 × 60 mm coverslips.

6. Incubate slides on a warming plate for 2–4 min at 75 °C (*see* **Note 8**).

7. Remove the coverslip immediately and place slide(s) in a Coplin jar filled with 70% ethanol (−20 °C; 3 min) to conserve target DNA as single strands.

8. Repeat **step 4**.

9. Use probe from **step 3** and add onto each denatured slide; put a suited coverslip on the drop and seal with rubber cement.

10. Incubate slides for 8–16 h at 37 °C in a humid chamber.

11. Take the slides out of the 37 °C chamber and remove the rubber cement and coverslips with forceps (optional: you can let them swim off in 1× SSC at RT, in a 100 ml Coplin jar).

12. Post-wash the slides 5 min in 1× SSC solution (62–64 °C) with gentle agitation.

13. Wash slides briefly in 1× PBS (at RT).

14. Dehydrate slides in an ethanol series (70%, 90%, and 100%, 3 min each) and air-dry.

15. Counterstain the slides with 20 μl of DAPI solution (antifade already included), cover with a coverslip 24 × 60, and evaluate the results under a fluorescence microscope (Fig. 1).

4   Notes

1. Blood or bone marrow treated with any anticoagulant can also be used. Sodium citrate-treated blood or bone marrow spreads the best.

2. Slides with smears can be used for up to 4 weeks after preparation if stored at 4 °C.

3. Before use, check culture media for possible contamination (color changes, cloudiness).

4. Sterile cell culture conditions must be maintained when handling living cells.

5. Remove supernatant off carefully with a glass pipette, 1 ml of supernatant can be left in the tube to avoid loss of material.

6. Denaturation of a probe can be done in water bath or, if available, more easily in a thermocycler.

7. Denatured (and prehybridized) probes should be applied to the denatured slide within 15–30 min; FISH can still be successful if applied after 60 min. Alternatively DNA probes and slides may be denatured simultaneously. However, not always denaturation time of probe and sample are alike and additionally common denaturation excludes prehybridization.

8. Denaturation times of only 2–4 min are suggested for the maintenance of available metaphase chromosomes. When heading for iFISH the time aspect is of no significance.

References

1. Jan M, Ebert BL, Jaiswal S (2017) Clonal hematopoiesis. Semin Hematol 54:43–50
2. Shanafelt TD (2009) Predicting clinical outcome in CLL: how and why. Hematology Am Soc Hematol Educ Program 2009:421–429
3. Bazargan A, Tam CS, Keating MJ (2012) Predicting survival in chronic lymphocytic leukemia. Expert Rev Anticancer Ther 12:393–403
4. Alhourani E, Rincic M, Othman MA, Pohle B, Schlie C, Glaser A et al (2014) Comprehensive chronic lymphocytic leukemia diagnostics by combined multiplex ligation dependent probe amplification (MLPA) and interphase fluorescence in situ hybridization (iFISH). Mol Cytogenet 7:79
5. Liehr T, Othman MA, Rittscher K, Alhourani E (2015) The current state of molecular cytogenetics in cancer diagnosis. Expert Rev Mol Diagn 15:517–526
6. Alhourani E, Aroutiounian R, Harutyunyan T, Glaser A, Schlie C, Pohle B et al (2016) Interphase molecular cytogenetic detection rates of chronic lymphocytic leukemia-specific aberrations are higher in cultivated cells than in blood or bone marrow smears. J Histochem Cytochem 64:495–501

Chapter 2

Detection of *RB1* Gene Copy Number Variations Using a Multiplex Ligation-Dependent Probe Amplification Method

Nejat Dalay

Abstract

Multiplex ligation-dependent probe amplification (MLPA) is based on simultaneous multiplex PCR of specific probes that hybridize to multiple different target DNA regions. The method can identify copy number changes, gross gene rearrangements, methylation patterns or even point mutations. MLPA has been a reliable approach to identify copy number changes in the clinical and research settings and is widely used for the screening and investigation of copy number variations and genomic aberrations of interest in various diseases. In this chapter the analysis of the copy number changes in the *RB1* gene locus by MLPA is described.

Key words Multiplex ligation-dependent probe amplification, Retinoblastoma protein, Copy number variation, Tumor suppressor genes, *RB1* gene

1 Introduction

Retinoblastoma is a malignant retinal childhood tumor with an estimated incidence of one case per 14,000–20,000 births. It is responsible for 1% of the deaths during childhood and the patients suffer from late complications resulting from the treatment [1]. The disease can be sporadic or hereditary. Sporadic retinoblastoma is caused by two independent somatic mutations in the retinal cells. In the hereditary cases a germ line mutation is derived from one of the parents. The mutations are transmitted in an autosomal dominant manner. Patients who carry the mutation have 90% risk of developing retinoblastoma and a 50% chance of transmitting the mutated gene to their offspring. All cases of bilateral retinoblastoma and approximately 10% of the patients with unilateral retinoblastoma are thought to carry a genetic predisposition. Inactivation of the normal *RB1* allele in the mutation carriers can occur by an additional mutation, loss of heterozygosity or promoter methylation. The hereditary form manifests itself at very early age with

Pedro G. Santiago-Cardona (ed.), *The Retinoblastoma Protein*, Methods in Molecular Biology, vol. 1726,
https://doi.org/10.1007/978-1-4939-7565-5_2, © Springer Science+Business Media, LLC 2018

bilateral and multifocal tumors. In bilateral tumors that are sporadic the germ line mutation is usually replaced by a de novo mutation in the germ cells at an early embryonic stage [2].

If detected at an early stage, the prognosis for retinoblastoma is very good. The survival is highest among the childhood cancers with 95% of the patients being cured. However, delay in the diagnosis and treatment increases the risk of nerve invasion, which is the most significant prognostic factor. Patients with hereditary retinoblastoma have also an increased risk of developing other types of cancers, including osteosarcomas, soft tissue sarcomas, and melanomas.

The *RB1* gene is located on chromosome 13q14. It consists of 27 exons and spans 183 kilobases. Several studies have shown common chromosomal alterations in retinoblastoma, including gains at chromosomes 1q, 2p, and 6p, and losses at 16q. More than 1500 alterations/mutations have been reported for the *RB1* gene [3]. These include a wide spectrum of deletions, point mutations, and insertions. Large rearrangements involving deletions and duplications of genomic regions act as an essential factor contributing to the development of tumors. Most of the alterations in the *RB1* gene result in the production of a truncated RB protein [4]. Recent studies have shown that family members of patients with hereditary retinoblastoma have an elevated risk of carrying the predisposing mutation and tumor development [5, 6]. Furthermore, the unaffected carriers can also transmit the mutation to their children. Therefore, detection of the predisposing mutations in the patients and families is of utmost importance. Identification of a germ line defect in a patient may guide the treatment helping clinical management and improving the outcome. It is also essential for the identification of relatives who carry a predisposing mutation and are at risk of developing cancers. Alternatively, exclusion of the genetic defect in a family member relieves noncarriers from regular examinations.

Advent of molecular diagnostic techniques and next generation sequencing have improved molecular screening of retinoblastoma. *RB1* gene testing is usually performed by analysis of the exons using direct sequencing and investigation of the copy number changes. Copy number variants (CNV) are structural gains or losses (deletions or duplications) compared to a reference genome ranging from 1 kb to several megabases. Since they affect a larger region of the genome they are an important component of genetic variation.

Although several different methods can be applied to the analysis of CNV, most of these are time-consuming and their sensitivity is low. Methods like FISH and karyotyping can only detect large deletions and rearrangements and have been replaced by more sensitive molecular methods. Multiplex ligation-dependent probe amplification (MLPA) is a fast and accurate sophisticated technology for copy number screening which combines the specificity of oligonucleotide hybridization with the advantages of PCR. Therefore, MLPA is an efficient method to analyze copy number variations in multiple samples with high precision on a common scale. The method is highly reproducible and is widely used to investigate genomic copy number changes for genetic analysis of various diseases [7–11]. In recent years, MLPA has been a preferred approach for the analysis of *RB1* gene deletions and duplications [12–17].

MLPA is a PCR-based method that allows detection of copy number changes at multiple different genomic loci simultaneously [18]. Up to 40–50 genomic regions or different genes can be analyzed in a single reaction [19]. MLPA allows rapid, accurate and reproducible screening of large numbers of samples for copy number changes in a single reaction, using a single primer pair. The most common application of MLPA is analysis of genomic aberrations but the method can also be adapted to various different applications, including analysis of point mutations, gene expression and methylation since MLPA can detect differences at a resolution level of a single nucleotide. The probes used in the MLPA assays are designed to recognize target sequences of 50–70 nucleotides. Therefore, even deletions of small target sequences or single exons on fragmented DNA can be analyzed.

The technique is based on the hybridization of two oligonucleotide half-probes to adjacent sides of target sequences. The two halves of the probes are then ligated. Only ligated probes can act as primers for the subsequent PCR reaction. Because the probes contain universal tails, the ligated probes can be amplified in a single reaction using a single primer pair. By this approach multiple target regions can be analyzed in a single assay. The 5′-ends of the primers used in the PCR are fluorescently labeled, allowing detection of the amplified fragments during separation by capillary electrophoresis. The probes used in a particular MLPA assay are designed to have different lengths. The unique length of each probe allows the detected signal to be easily associated with the corresponding probe. The resulting signal is proportional to the amount of the target sequences in the sample and the relative differences in the peak heights reflect the variations in the copy numbers. Using MLPA copy number changes of up to 50 specific genomic regions can be investigated in the clinical setting.

MLPA kits usually contain 40–50 different probes usually targeting exonic sequences of the genes. The number of the probes used for each individual assay depends on the aim of the study. Several reference probes are included in the assay that are directed against chromosomal regions in which copy number variations are not observed. The signals from each of the probes in the MLPA reaction are easily identified by their typical length. The relative signals from the samples are compared to the signals from the reference probes to determine the peak height ratios for the region of interest. These signals are proportional to the number of the target sequences present for the corresponding probe in the sample. However, to translate the data into copy numbers, the signal intensity of each probe from the sample is compared with the corresponding signal from the reference sample.

2 Materials

The reagents required for performing MLPA analysis are obtained from MRC Holland (Netherlands), the sole provider of the MLPA kits and the probemixes. The components found in the typical reaction kit are indicated below, additional reagents not provided in the kits can be purchased from different suppliers. The probemixes needed for each particular assay are ordered separately. MRC Holland has probemixes for a variety of different applications which can be used depending on the aim of the study. The probemix 047-D1 RB1 has been specifically designed to detect copy number variations in the *RB1* gene as well as methylation of the *RB1* gene promoter, thus, all reagents and procedures described in this chapter refer to the 047-D1 RB1 probemix used to detect copy number variations in the *RB1* locus. Alternative kits for more general applications which contain several probes for the *RB1* gene are also available (Table 1), protocols for the MLPA assays using different probemixes are available at the MRC Holland website (www.mlpa.com). Alternatively, custom MLPA probes targeting unique sequences can also be designed (*see* **Note 1**). However, most frequently the 047-D1 RB1 probemix is used for analysis of the *RB1* copy number variations. The probemix contains 36 probes recognizing 26 exons of the *RB1* gene, 13 different reference probes, and 7 flanking probes for assessing the presence of copy number changes.

The vials in the MLPA kit containing different reagents are characterized by caps with different colors, and are listed below.

2.1 Reagents Found in the SALSA MLPA Kit (See Note 2)

The SALSA MLPA EK kits are available for 100 (EK1) or 500 (EK5) reactions and with appropriate labels for use with the ABI (FAM) or Beckman (Cy5) platforms.

1. SALSA MLPA Buffer.

2. SALSA Ligase-65 Enzyme.

3. Ligase buffer A.

4. Ligase buffer B.

5. SALSA PCR Primer mix (*see* **Note 3**).

6. SALSA Polymerase.

7. SALSA MLPA Probe Mix. This is the SALSA MLPA 047-D1 RB1 Probemix, which is sold separately. These probemix kits are also available in different sizes for 25, 50, or 100 reactions.

Table 1
MLPA probemixes containing probes for the *RB1* gene

Name of the probemix	Number of probes	Size of the probes	Location
ME 002	2	319	354 nt before exon 1
		472	157 nt before exon 1
P 146-B1	1	459	Exon 26
P 294-B1	2	401	Exon 3
		488	Exon 25
P 335-B2	5	220	Exon 6
		315	Exon 14
		358	Exon 19
		418	Exon 24
		445	Exon 26
P 377	2	469	Exon 23
		489	Exon 27
P 425	2	250	Exon 8
		454	Exon 26

2.2 Reagents and Equipment Not Included in the Kit

1. Dye-labeled DNA size Standard (CEQ or Genescan) for use in the analysis by capillary electrophoresis (Subheading 3.3, **step 1**). CEQ and Genescan are the labeled DNA size standards for capillary electrophoresis when using the Beckman or ABI systems, respectively. The Genescan 500 kit contains 16 fragments ranging from 35 to 500 nucleotides and the CEQ Size Standard 600 kit includes 33 fragments ranging from 60 to 640 nucleotides. When a system from a different capillary electrophoresis manufacturer is used, a corresponding size standard suitable for this particular instrument should be selected.

2. TE Buffer: 10 mM Tris–HCl, pH 8.2, 0.1 mM EDTA.

3. Hi-Di Formamide.

4. POP-4 polymer for genetic analyzers.

5. LIZ GeneScan 500 (or ROX GeneScan 500) Size Standard. LIZ-labeled standards are preferable when using ABI systems to prevent spectral overlaps.

6. Thermal cycler with heated lid, with corresponding PCR tubes (*see* **Note 4**).

7. Capillary electrophoresis system (ABI Prism Genetic Analyzer).

8. Genemapper (ABI) or GeneMarker (Softgenetics, LLC) software.

3 Methods

3.1 Preparation and Isolation of DNA

The results of the MLPA analysis depend heavily on the quality of the DNA samples (*see* **Note 5**). No specific DNA extraction protocol is necessary as long as the procedure yields DNA of satisfactory quality. The MRC-Holland website states that their methods have been tested using the Qiagen Autopure LS, QIAamp DNA, or Promega DNA Extraction Wizard kits, however, the methods described below work well even with standard protocols for DNA extraction. Degradation of DNA can in some instances lead to erroneous results when analyzing copy numbers. However, MLPA has the advantage that even if the extracted DNA has been subjected to some degradation due to different factors, copy number analysis by MLPA can usually be performed successfully since the probes used in the assay target relatively short DNA sequences of 50–80 bp (*see* **Note 6**). The purity and concentration of the genomic DNA samples are also very important (*see* **Note 7**).

3.2 MLPA Assay

Detailed protocols for each individual MLPA assay using specific probe mixes are available at the MRC Holland website (*see* **Note 8**). The MLPA assay protocol described in this section refers to the 047-D1 RB1 probemix. Regarding steps that involve water, the MLPA protocol suggests the use of ultrapure water, but in our experience PCR-grade water works equally well.

1. Thaw buffers and probemix and vortex before use.

2. Dissolve 5 μl of DNA sample (50–100 ng) in TE buffer in a PCR tube/microplate well (*see* **Note 9**).

3. Denature the samples in the thermocycler at 98 °C for 5 min and allow them to come to room temperature before removing from the thermocycler (*see* **Note 10**).

4. To each sample add 3 μl mix containing 1.5 μl SALSA MLPA Probemix and 1.5 μl SALSA MLPA buffer.

5. Mix and incubate in the thermocycler at 95 °C for 1 min and at 60 °C for 16 h.

6. To prepare the "ligase mix," add 25 μl H_2O, 3 μl of Ligase buffer A and 3 μl Ligase buffer B to a tube, mix gently and add 1 μl SALSA Ligase 65 enzyme, mix again (Do not vortex! *see* **Note 11**).

7. Bring the thermocycler from 60 to 54 °C and add 32 μl of the ligase mix into each tube without removing the samples from the thermocycler. Mix gently, do not use vortex.

8. Perform ligation by incubating in the thermocycler at 54 °C for 15 min.

9. Inactivate the ligase for 5 min at 98 °C. Then let the samples cool to 20 °C. (At this point the tubes can be removed from the thermocycler).

10. Prepare the necessary amount of the Polymerase Master Mix by adding 7.5 μl H_2O, 2 μl SALSA PCR primer mix and 0.5 μl SALSA polymerase for each reaction. Mix well before use. Do not vortex! (*see* **Note 12**).

11. Add 10 μl Polymerase Master Mix to each tube, mix gently by pipetting. Do not vortex!

12. Place the tubes in the thermocycler and run the PCR reaction as follows (*see* **Note 13**):

35 cycles of	30 s at 90 °C
	30 s at 60 °C
	60 s at 72 °C
	Final incubation for 20 min at 72 °C

13. Cool the mixture to room temperature (*see* **Note 14**).

3.3 Analysis by Capillary Electrophoresis

Separation and analysis of the fragments is performed using capillary electrophoresis. Any type of modern standard capillary electrophoresis system can be used for analysis. The experimental conditions, reactants, components and parameters may differ depending on the type of instrument used. The MRC Holland website provides detailed instructions for the experimental setup and instrument settings to be used when using different ABI Prism or Beckman systems (*see* **Note 15**). This section describes the conditions used for the ABI Prism (3100, 3130, 3730) instruments which have been validated for use with the MRC Holland MLPA products. When using these instruments, FAM is used as the fluorescent label for the primers and POP-4 is the preferred polymer for separation. Thirty-six or 50 cm capillaries (for ABI 3500 only 50 cm) can be used for analysis. For details on the use of different systems and conditions to be used with other instruments consult the instructions of the instrument manufacturer and the MRC Holland website (MLPA procedure).

1. Mix 0.7 μl of each PCR reaction product with 0.2 μl LIZ GeneScan 500 size Standard (or alternatively, 0.3 μl of ROX GeneScan 500) and 9 μl Hi-Di Formamide (*see* **Note 16**).

2. Denature at 86 °C for 3 min, cool at 4 °C for 2 min, then bring to room temperature.

3. Analyze by capillary electrophoresis (*see* **Note 17**).

3.4 Analysis of the Results

Analysis of raw data includes the recognition of the peaks and assigning of these signals with the corresponding targets before comparative analysis (Fig. 1). During this step the quality of the available data for each sample is evaluated. Problems due to incomplete separation, artifacts from the PCR reaction, stutter bands, etc. are inspected and corrections or adjustments are made when necessary. For the visualization of the peak patterns and detecting the peak intensities the Genemapper (ABI) or GeneMarker (Softgenetics, LLC) software can be used. The integrated peak areas can be exported to an Excel-based spreadsheet using these software for further analysis. Alternatively, the Coffalyzer software (MRC Holland) can be used for quality control and to perform the complete analysis. The Coffalyzer software is a freeware which can be downloaded from the MRC Holland website. All files generated by the ABI or Beckman (CEQ) capillary electrophoresis systems are directly recognized and read by the Coffalyzer software. Genemapper data can also be directly exported to the Coffalyzer software for normalization of raw data and copy number analysis.

3.4.1 MLPA Quality Control Fragments

Each MLPA reaction contains several quality control fragments which help to determine whether the quantity of DNA used in the experiment is sufficient, the ligation is successful or denaturation is complete (*see* **Note 18**). Consult the information on the use of the corresponding kits and probe mixes at the MRC Holland website for evaluation and interpretation of the peaks from the quality control fragments provided in the kit.

3.4.2 Normalization

The peaks generated by the capillary electrophoresis analysis reflect the absolute fluorescence values. During the PCR amplification different probes may display different amplification efficiencies depending on the sequence of the probe. This may lead to differences in the amplification of the references and samples. Therefore, the data need to be normalized to determine the relative peak heights before further analysis. This is necessary to prevent possible abnormal readings from the reference probes affecting the results. The normalization process is achieved in two steps. Intrasample normalization normalizes the peak areas from the individual probes with respect to the peak areas of the reference probes for all samples, while intersample normalization is achieved by normalization of each individual sample versus the normal reference DNA from the control subjects. During the first step (intrasample normalization) the height of the peak from each probe is compared to the height of every reference probe resulting in multiple ratios (as many as the number of the reference probes) and then the median value of these ratios is determined. This value is used as the normalization constant for this particular probe when comparing the samples to the references.

Intersample normalization is used to compare each test sample to the corresponding control sample to determine the ploidy status. This is accomplished by dividing the intranormalized probe ratio from each probe in the patient sample by the average (median) intranormalized probe ratio of all reference samples from the controls for that probe. The normalized final results show the difference between the signal intensities of the sample and the references.

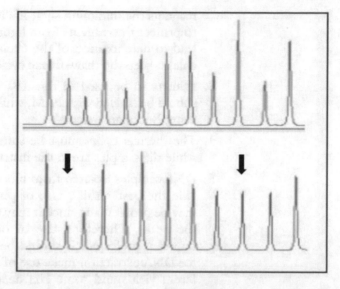

Fig. 1 Representative peaks from capillary electrophoresis of the amplification products for copy number analysis. The vertical axis depicts the fluorescence signal reflecting the amount of the corresponding fragment and the horizontal axis represents the fragment length (in nucleotides). Note the decreased height of peaks 2 and 10 in the lower sample. Peaks from each individual sample (reference and patient) need first to be normalized within the sample, (e.g., the peak area from the corresponding probe should be compared to the mean peak areas of the all reference probes for that sample) and then the final probe ratio is determined by comparing this value to the corresponding value for the same peak from the reference samples. A final ratio < 0.7 or >1.3 indicate deletions or duplications, respectively. These steps of the analysis are best performed by exporting data to the Coffalyzer software

For normal diploid loci the normalized probe ratio is expected to be 1.0. A deviation of 30% is usually accepted as the cutoff threshold to indicate a deletion or duplication [20]. Probe ratios less than 0.7 are considered deletions and values higher than 1.3 are regarded as duplications.

4 Notes

1. When designing custom reference probes it should be noted that these need to target and hybridize to variation-free DNA regions. The right hemiprobe (right half) of each oligonucleotide probe should be phosphorylated at the 5′-end for ligation to occur. To adjust the length of the probes for easy identification stuffer sequences of varying length may be introduced when necessary.

2. The reagents in the SALSA MLPA kit should be stored in the freezer at −20 °C in their original package. For properly stored

reagents the minimum shelf-life is 1 year. Care must be taken to protect the reagents from light. Thawing and freezing may lead to deterioration of the chemicals. Therefore, it is advisable to keep the thaw–freeze cycles as low as possible.

3. Primers to be used in the ABI Biosystem genetic analyzers should be labeled with FAM, while Cy5 is the label for analysis using Beckman systems.

4. The thermal cycler must be suitable for adding the reagents while the samples are in the instrument.

5. DNA samples isolated from blood or fresh tumor tissue provide the best results. Use of phenol during DNA isolation may be problematic since it may distort the signals and affect the peaks. Therefore, use of other DNA extraction techniques is preferred. It should be noted that commercial kits for DNA extraction make use of different methods, have different yields and some kits need an additional purification step before MLPA can be performed. Different extraction methods may affect the relative peak heights and can lead to unreliable data suggesting copy number differences. Therefore, all samples used in the assay should be isolated by the same procedure.

6. When paraffin-embedded tissue is used the quality of the DNA may cause problems. The quality of the DNA samples isolated from paraffin blocks may be low, DNA can be fragmented or denatured due to formalin treatment and may harbor structural alterations. The fixation process may also affect DNA quality. The type of the fixative, as well as the duration, pH, or temperature of the fixation procedure, plays a role in the quality of the DNA sample. Extremely short or long fixation periods are known to increase the number of the peak intensities beyond the normal range affecting the calculations [21].

7. Too high concentrations should not be used since they may induce signals outside of the proportional signal range.

8. During the MLPA assay keep all solutions and reagents on ice. When preparing reagent mixes it is advisable to add 5–10% surplus volume for easy pipetting.

9. The amount of DNA used in the MLPA can be as low as 20 ng. The reaction mixture should contain 5–10 mM TE buffer to avoid DNA damage.

10. Incomplete denaturation of DNA can restrict probe binding. Allow sufficient time for complete denaturation.

11. Never vortex enzyme solutions! If the enzyme solution is mixed too violently the enzyme may be inactivated. However, if the enzyme solution is not perfectly mixed with the buffer

this may also lead to inaccurate results. The mixes and solutions containing enzymes should be mixed gently by pipetting. Prepare the ligase and polymerase master mixes less than 1/2 h before pipetting and keep on ice.

12. When preparing the master mixes always add the enzymes last. Warm the tube containing the SALSA polymerase enzyme in the hand for 5–10 s before adding the enzyme to tubes. Perform this procedure while keeping the tubes on ice. Since the dyes used to label the primers are light-sensitive take also care that exposure of the primers to light is minimized during these steps.

13. Any contamination during the PCR reaction may result in aberrant signals which can be interpreted as false positive results. Therefore, care should be taken to prevent contamination during PCR. Analysis of the samples in duplicate can help to overcome these artifacts. Residual phenol, ethanol, and TRIzol, high salt or presence of metal ions may lead to variations in the MLPA results.

14. The PCR products can be stored in the refrigerator for up to 1 week. If longer storage is needed the products are stable in the freezer at −20 °C.

15. To achieve the best separation performance the instrument settings usually need some optimization. Familiarize yourself with the performance characteristics of the system in use. Consult the manufacturer's instructions when adjusting the specific instrument parameters.

16. It may be necessary to adjust the amount of the PCR product to obtain the best peaks. Note that adding more product to the injection mixture adversely affects the separation by increasing the salt concentration. If the peak heights are not satisfactory try increasing the injection time or the voltage instead of adding more PCR product.

17. Use of old, previously used capillaries or polymers may have adverse effects on the results. This results in lower peak heights and in some broadening of the peaks from the size standards. Change the polymer and capillaries at regular intervals. The polymer undergoes degradation and loses its capacity when exposed to temperatures higher than 25 °C.

18. The four Q-fragments indicate the amount of the DNA sample used in the test and the results of the ligation reaction. Normally peaks from these fragments should be at least 5–10 times lower when compared to the peaks from the probes. Higher peaks comparable to those from the probes indicate low sample DNA or poor ligation. Low peaks from the D-(denaturation) fragments indicate incomplete denaturation.

References

1. Kivelä T (2009) 200 years of success initiated by James Wardrop's 1809 monograph on retinoblastoma. Acta Ophthalmol 87:810–812

2. Lohmann DR, Gallie BL (2004) Retinoblastoma: revisiting the model prototype of inherited cancer. Am J Med Genet 129C:23–28

3. Leiden Open Variation Database. http://rb1-lovd.d-lohmann.de/home.php?select_db=RB1. Accessed 15 Feb 2017

4. Harbour JW (1998) Overview of RB gene mutations in patients with retinoblastoma. Implications for clinical genetic screening. Ophthalmology 105:1442–1447

5. MacCarthy A, Bayne AM, Brownbill PA et al (2013) Second and subsequent tumours among 1927 retinoblastoma patients diagnosed in Britain 1951–2004. Br J Cancer 108:2455–2463

6. Kleinerman RA, Yu CL, Little MP et al (2012) Variation of second cancer risk by family history of retinoblastoma among long-term survivors. J Clin Oncol 30:950–957

7. Hömig-Hölzel C, Savola S (2012) Multiplex ligation-dependent probe amplification (MLPA) in tumor diagnostics and prognostics. Diagn Mol Pathol 21:189–206

8. Aoyama Y, Yamamoto T, Sakaguchi N et al (2015) Application of multiplex ligation-dependent probe amplification, and identification of a heterozygous Alu-associated deletion and a uniparental disomy of chromosome 1 in two patients with 3-hydroxy-3-methylglutaryl-CoA lyase deficiency. Int J Mol Med 35:1554–1560

9. Zauber P, Marotta S, Sabbath-Solitare M (2016) Copy number of the Adenomatous Polyposis Coli gene is not always neutral in sporadic colorectal cancers with loss of heterozygosity for the gene. BMC Cancer 16:213

10. Wang J, Ai X, Qin T et al (2017) Multiplex ligation-dependent probe amplification assay identifies additional copy number changes compared with R-band karyotype and provide more accuracy prognostic information in myelodysplastic syndromes. Oncotarget 8:1603–1612

11. Yalniz Z, Demokan S, Karabulut B et al (2017) Copy number profiling of tumor suppressor genes in head and neck cancer. Head Neck 39:341–346

12. Price EA, Price K, Kolkiewicz K et al (2014) Spectrum of RB1 mutations identified in 403 retinoblastoma patients. J Med Genet 51:208–214

13. Dommering CJ, Mol BM, Moll AC et al (2014) RB1 mutation spectrum in a comprehensive nationwide cohort of retinoblastoma patients. J Med Genet 51:366–374

14. He MY, An Y, Gao YJ et al (2016) Screening of RB1 gene mutations in Chinese patients with retinoblastoma and preliminary exploration of genotype-phenotype correlations. Mol Vis 20:545–552

15. Shahraki K, Ahani A, Sharma P et al (2016) Genetic screening in Iranian patients with retinoblastoma. Eye (Lond) 31:620–627

16. Ahani A, Akbari MT, Saliminejad K et al (2013) Screening for large rearrangements of the RB1 gene in Iranian patients with retinoblastoma using multiplex ligation-dependent probe amplification. Mol Vis 19:454–462

17. Khalid MKNM, Yakob Y, Yasin RM et al (2015) Spectrum of germ-line RB1 gene mutations in Malaysian patients with retinoblastoma. Mol Vis 21:1185–1190

18. Schouten JP, McElgunn CJ, Waaijer R et al (2002) Relative quantification of 40 nucleic acid sequences by multiplex ligation-dependent probe amplification. Nucleic Acids Res 30:e57

19. Nygren AO, Ameziane N, Duarte HM et al (2005) Methylation-specific MLPA (MS-MLPA): simultaneous detection of CpG methylation and copy number changes of up to 40 sequences. Nucleic Acids Res 33:e128

20. Bunyan DJ, Eccles DM, Sillibourne J et al (2004) Dosage analysis of cancer predisposition genes by multiplex ligation-dependent probe amplification. Br J Cancer 91:1155–1159

21. Atanesyan L, Steenkamer MJ, Horstman A et al (2017) Optimal fixation conditions and DNA extraction methods for MLPA analysis on FFPE tissue-derived DNA. Am J Clin Pathol 41:1443–1455

Chapter 3

A Fluorescent Quantitative Multiplex PCR Method to Detect Copy Number Changes in the *RB1* Gene

Chitra Kannabiran

Abstract

Copy number changes comprising deletions or insertions involving single or multiple exons of a gene are known to occur in a significant proportion of cases in retinoblastoma. The protocol described here involves a two-step quantitative multiplex PCR process which is suitable for the detection of such mutations in the RB1 as well as in other genes. This is achieved through the use of suitable gene-specific primers designed to amplify individual exons, with universal tags attached to the 5′ end of each primer. These tagged primers are used in the first step of PCR of the RB1 gene in patients. The second step is carried out through the use of "universal" primers complementary to the tag sequences alone. This technique facilitates the detection of fluorescent PCR products from multiple exons through the use of a single fluorescent tagged primer.

Key words RB1, Quantitative PCR, Multiplex PCR, Fluorescent tags, Copy number, Deletion, Insertion

1 Introduction

The *RB1* gene (GenBank accession L11910.1; cDNA L41870.1) is located on chromosome 13q14 and is disrupted by mutations in retinoblastoma and other types of cancers. The gene is about 180 kilobases in length, and consists of 27 exons, encoding a transcript of 4.6 kb. The encoded protein (pRb) is 928 amino acids long. Two mutational events in the *RB1* gene are involved in the development of retinoblastoma as postulated by the two-hit theory of oncogenesis by Knudson [1]. Retinoblastomas can be either hereditary or nonhereditary. In the former type, one allele of the *RB1* gene is mutated in the germ line (therefore detectable in constitutional cells of the affected individual), and the second allele is mutated in the developing retinal tissue. In the nonhereditary form, both alleles of the *RB1* gene undergo somatic mutations (in the retinal cells). Thus, though the inheritance of the disease follows a dominant pattern, occurring by the transmission of one mutant allele of *RB1* through the germ line, the development of the tumor

Pedro G. Santiago-Cardona (ed.), *The Retinoblastoma Protein*, Methods in Molecular Biology, vol. 1726,
https://doi.org/10.1007/978-1-4939-7565-5_3, © Springer Science+Business Media, LLC 2018

follows a recessive pattern, since mutation of the second allele (or the second hit) occurs at the cellular level, and mutations of both alleles are required for the disease to manifest. The majority of patients with retinoblastoma show sporadic cases, having no affected family members. About 10% of patients have familial disease. However, all patients with bilateral retinoblastoma and about 10–12% of unilateral sporadic cases are germ cell mutants, implying that even if they present as sporadic cases, they carry germ line *RB1* mutations that can be transmitted to their offspring. The remaining 88–90% of cases of unilateral retinoblastoma are nonhereditary.

Identification of mutations in *RB1* in affected children is clinically useful in genetic testing and predicting the risk of disease in offspring and relatives of patients. Stepwise approaches to testing for different types of mutations have been developed by combining a battery of molecular techniques designed to detect all types of mutations ranging from copy number changes to point mutations and hyper-methylation. With an optimized sensitivity of detection, testing of immediate family members of probands can reveal mutation carriers and thus inform clinical management of the family [2]. Application of the test in prenatal diagnosis can lead to early and more effective treatment for individuals who are positive for a *RB1* gene mutation. In fact, preimplantation genetic diagnosis (PGD) has been applied to detect *RB1* mutations in embryos. Single cell analysis on embryos obtained by in vitro fertilization with intracytoplasmic sperm injection has been successfully used for detection of the *RB1* mutation present on the paternal allele. This allowed the selection of embryos that were free of the mutation, for implantation into the uterus [3]. Knowing the *RB1* mutational status in the probands and their immediate family members may help in the avoidance of unnecessary clinical examinations of relatives who are noncarriers of *RB1* mutations and therefore not at risk of developing malignant tumors. Thus, one of the potential benefits of *RB1* gene testing is that it can lead to savings in costs incurred in the clinic.

RB1 mutations occurring in retinoblastoma range from single base changes (point mutations), to large deletions affecting the entire gene and resulting in copy number changes such as hemizygosity due to deletion of one allele of the *RB1* gene. These mutations are distributed throughout the length of the gene, and all exons except the last two, are involved. Based on consequence of mutations, over 90% of all mutations in *RB1* represent null mutations. Data compiled from studies in several populations indicate that about one-third or more of patients have frameshift mutations, an equal proportion have nonsense mutations, one-third or less have splice mutations and up to 10% of cases generally have missense mutations [4]. Based on the size and types of mutation, about 50% or more of *RB1* mutations are point mutations (affecting single bases) including nonsense, missense and splice site mutations, about 20% are small length mutations (deletions or insertions or a few bases), and 10–20% are large deletions [5, 6]. Among the point mutations which affect a single base, transitions affecting CpG dinucleotides are recurrent features in the *RB1* mutational spectrum and result in conversion of CGA (Arg) to TGA (Stop) codons, with premature termination. In particular, 12 arginine codons have been identified as sites of highly recurrent mutations, accounting for over 75% of all recurrent mutations in RB1 [2].

From the foregoing, it is evident that the *RB1* gene shows extensive mutational heterogeneity, and multiple techniques capable of detecting the entire range of mutations are required to achieve the complete detection of oncogenic mutations for clinical genetic testing. While routine PCR amplification and sequencing are sufficient for the detection of point mutations and small deletions or insertions (of a few bases), the identification of large deletions or insertions particularly in heterozygous patients, has been routinely done using other methods. These include quantitative PCR, MLPA (*m*ultiplex *l*igation-dependent *p*robe *a*mplification), real-time PCR, and more recently, next generation sequencing technology.

We have developed a combinatorial approach designed to detect different types of mutations in *RB1*, being able to achieve detection rates of 80% or more [6]. For detecting large deletions/ insertions, we employed a form of quantitative multiplex PCR adapted from a protocol termed universal primer quantitative fluorescent multiplex (UPQFM) PCR, described by Heath and coworkers [7]. In this technique, different exon-specific primers are tagged with a common sequence at the 5'end of both forward and reverse primers. These "tag" sequences are separate for forward and reverse primers, with a single tag sequence being common to all forward primers or all reverse primers. In addition, the protocol as modified in our laboratory includes an internal control in the UPQFM PCR reactions, which is a PCR product of an exon of a gene on a different chromosome than *RB1*. We used the exon 6 of beta-IGH3 (β-IGH3; TGFBI, transforming growth factor beta-induced) gene on chromosome 5. Thus, the primers for the internal control have the same tag sequences as the *RB1* primers, and are included in all multiplex reactions.

Quantitative PCR is carried out in two steps—the first step amplifies the *RB1* exons from the DNA templates provided, with primers that have the *RB1* gene-specific sequences attached to a common 'tag' sequence at the 5' end. The tag sequences for forward and reverse primers are 5'-TCCGTCTTAGCTGAGTGGCGT-3' (forward primer) and 5'-ACCTCTGGGTAATGGAATTATTATT-3' (reverse primer). The first PCR is carried out for 10–15 cycles and the reactions are stopped at this stage, an aliquot is removed from each reaction, and used as template for the second PCR. In the second stage, the primers are specific to the tag sequences only, and are therefore termed as "universal primers" as they can amplify PCR products from any gene, provided they are flanked by the same tag sequences.

2 Materials

2.1 Genomic DNA Extraction Reagents

Stock reagents for extraction of genomic DNA were prepared exactly as described by Sambrook et al. [8].

1. Phosphate-buffered saline (PBS): the standard recipe for 1 L of 1× PBS consists of 8 g NaCl, 0.2 g KCl, 1.44 g Na_2HPO_4, and 0.24 g KH_2PO_4. Dissolve in 800 mL H_2O, adjust pH to 7.4 with HCl, and complete final volume of 1 L with H_2O. Dispense into aliquots and sterilize either by autoclaving (20 min at 15 PSI) or by filtering.

2. 1 M Tris–HCl buffer, pH 8.0: Dissolve 121.1 g of Tris base in 800 mL of H_2O. Adjust the pH to 8.0 with HCl.

3. Lysis buffer: 0.5% SDS, 0.1 M EDTA, and 10 mM Tris–HCl, pH 8.0.

4. 0.5 M ethylene diamine tetra-acetic acid (EDTA): To prepare add 186.1 g of disodium EDTA·$2H_2O$ to 800 mL of H_2O. Stir vigorously on a magnetic stirrer. Adjust the pH to 8.0 with NaOH (~20 g of NaOH pellets). Dispense into aliquots and sterilize by autoclaving. The disodium salt of EDTA will not go into solution until the pH of the solution is adjusted to ~8.0 by the addition of NaOH.

5. 10% sodium dodecyl sulfate (SDS): Dissolve 10 g of SDS in 80 mL of H_2O, and then add H_2O to 100 mL. This stock solution is stable for 6 months at room temperature.

6. Proteinase K, RNAse.

7. Saturated phenol (saturated with 0.1 M Tris–HCl, pH 8.0).

8. Chloroform.

9. 10 M ammonium acetate: To prepare a 10 M solution in 1 L, dissolve 770 g of ammonium acetate in 800 mL of H_2O. Adjust volume to 1 L with H_2O. Sterilize by filtration. Alternatively, to prepare a 100-mL solution, dissolve 77 g of ammonium acetate in 70 mL of H_2O at room temperature. Adjust the volume to 100 mL with H_2O. Sterilize the solution by passing it through a 0.22-μm filter. Store the solution in tightly sealed bottles at 4 °C or at room temperature. Ammonium acetate decomposes in hot H_2O and solutions containing it should not be autoclaved.

10. Tris–EDTA (TE) buffer: 10 mM Tris–HCl pH 8.0, 2 mM EDTA.

11. Ethanol 70% and 95%.

2.2 Primer Sets	Primers, labeled with 6-FAM, as well as unlabeled, must be custom synthesized and ordered from commercial suppliers.

1. RB1 gene specific primers. These primers should have universal tags at 5'end of both forward and reverse primers. *See* Table 1 for examples of RB1 gene specific primers.

2. Tag-specific Primers. These are complementary only to each of the forward and reverse tag sequences. One of the tag-specific primers should be labeled with a fluorescent dye, such as 6-Fam, that is compatible with the detection system of the ABI genetic analyzer (Applied Biosystems Incorporated).

2.3   PCR Reagents

1. 25 mM magnesium chloride ($MgCl_2$).

2. Standard 10× PCR buffer.

3. Taq polymerase.

4. 10 mM deoxynucleoside triphosphates (dNTPs).

2.4   Equipment, Software, and Labware

1. ABI3130XL system.

2. Routine glassware and disposable plasticware including microfuge tubes 1.5 mL, 0.5 mL, and PCR tubes of 0.2 mL volume. Tips for pipettors (10, 200, and 1000 μL) are required.

3. Table top microcentrifuge.

4. Spectrophotometer.

5. Thermal cycler.

6. ABI Genetic Analyzer system.

Table 1
Examples of *RB1* gene specific primers with universal tags at 5′ end of both forward and reverse primers

Primer	Sequence	Amplicon size
5 (F)	<u>TCCGTCTTAGCTGAGTGGCGTA</u>TTGGGAAAATCTACTTGAACTTTG	340
5 (R)	<u>AGGCAGAATCGACTCACCGCT</u>AGCTATAATCGATCAAACTAACCCT	
6 (F)	<u>TCCGTCTTAGCTGAGTGGCGTA</u>TTTTTCCTGTTTTTTTTCTGCTTTCT	222
6 (R)	<u>AGGCAGAATCGACTCACCGCTA</u>ATTTAGTCCAAAGGAATGCCAA	
7 (F)	<u>TCCGTCTTAGCTGAGTGGCGTA</u>CCTGCGATTTTCTCTCATACAA	284
7 (R)	<u>AGGCAGAATCGACTCACCGCTA</u>AGACATTCAATAAGCAACTGCTGA	
Uni-F	6-Fam-<u>TCCGTCTTAGCTGAGTGGCGTA</u>	
Uni-R	<u>AGGCAGAATCGACTCACCGCTA</u>	

Primers are designated with the corresponding exon numbers and forward (F) or reverse (R). Tags are underlined. Uni-F and Uni-R denote universal primers that are specific for tag sequences of forward and reverse primers, respectively. One of the universal primers is labeled with 6-Fam

7. GeneScan™ 500 LIZ™ dye Size Standard.

8. Gene Mapper software (Applied Biosystems Incorporated.)

---

3 Methods

3.1 DNA Preparation

We routinely prepare genomic DNA by the method described below. However, you can use any standard method for genomic DNA extraction from blood leukocytes. Regardless of the methods, you need to check the quality of DNA by spectrophotometry at 260 and 280 nm. A A260/A280 ratio of about 1.8 is recommended for reliable results.

1. Thaw frozen blood samples (~4–5 mL each), and mix with an equal volume of PBS.

2. Centrifuge at 3500 rpm in a benchtop centrifuge for 10 min to get a leukocyte pellet.

3. Suspend the pellet in lysis buffer and treat with proteinase K (100 µg/mL) and RNase (20 µg/mL).

4. Extract the lysate with an equal volume of saturated phenol (pH 8.0), phenol–chloroform mix, and then with chloroform.

5. Remove the aqueous phase, and precipitate the DNA by adding one-fifth volume of 10 M ammonium acetate, and two volumes of 95% ethanol. DNA may be removed by spooling on to a glass Pasteur pipette, and then transferred to a microfuge tube.

6. Wash the DNA precipitate with 70% ethanol, followed by centrifugation at 10,000 rpm in a benchtop centrifuge for 15 min. Drain the pellet to remove the ethanol, and allow it to air dry. Resuspend the pellet in TE buffer.

7. Estimate the concentration and purity of DNA by spectrophotometry, and make working dilutions of 20–50 ng/µL for PCR reactions from stock DNA solutions.

3.2 PCR Reactions

Set up PCR reactions in a designated area that is used only for PCR set-up, separate from genomic DNA preparation or gel electrophoresis. Pipettors, plasticware, and reagents used for setting up PCR reactions should be kept separate from those used for post-PCR work. Use autoclaved plasticware for setting up reactions. Use standard 0.2 mL PCR tubes or plates. All PCR reagents used in this section are standard and available from many commercial suppliers. Primers are reconstituted in de-ionized, autoclaved water, as per the amounts indicated in the product information sheet from the manufacturers. Stock primers are generally diluted to a concentration of 100 pmol/µL. Working solutions of primers for use in PCR reactions are made by dilution of stock primers to 5 or 10 pmol/µL. These reagents are stored in aliquots at −20 °C.

There are two PCR reactions performed on every template, the P1 and P2 reactions.

3.2.1 P1 PCR Reaction

Conduct the P1 reaction using the tagged exonic primers in a multiplex PCR reaction to amplify DNA from patients or controls. Design primers having the common 'tag' sequences at the 5′ end followed by test gene-specific sequences (in this case RB1) for each of the forward and reverse primers. You also need to select a suitable gene as internal control, in addition to the 'test' gene to be evaluated, located on a different chromosome. Design primers for amplification of any one of the exons of the internal control as well, having the same tag sequences as the test gene. Limit the size of PCR products to be amplified to 350 bp or less (*see* **Notes 1** and **2**).

1. Thaw DNA samples and all frozen reagents including primers, deoxynucleoside triphosphates (dNTPs), magnesium chloride, and 10× PCR buffer on the bench.

2. Mix each reagent after thawing on a vortexer or by a short spin on a centrifuge. Genomic DNA may be pipetted up and down to mix, or vortexed at low speed to avoid fragmentation.

3. Set the P1 reactions as follows in a 20 μL volume: 20–50 ng genomic DNA, 5 pmol each of forward and reverse primers, $MgCl_2$ to a concentration of 1.5 mM, dNTPs to a concentration of 200 μM, 2 μL of 10× PCR buffer, and 1–2 units of Taq polymerase. Add deionized water to bring the reaction mixture to 20 μL total volume (*see* **Notes 3** and **4**).

4. Carry out the P1 PCR reactions for a limited number of cycles (between 10 and 15 cycles), so that PCR is in the exponential phase.

5. Stop the P1 reaction, and take an aliquot of the P1 reaction and use it as a template for the second PCR, which is the P2 PCR described in the next section.

3.2.2 P2 PCR Reaction

Conduct PCR reaction 2 using the universal primers that bind to the tag sequences present in P1 amplicons. All components in the P2 reactions are the same as in P1 except the primers and template (*see* **Note 3**).

1. Set up the following PCR reaction: to each reaction, add 5 pmol each of Uni-F and Uni-R primers and 2 μL of P1 reaction mix as template. Complete the volume to 20 μL with dH_2O.

3.3 Electrophoresis of Samples on ABI Genetic Analyzer

Reagents for the ABI Genetic analyzer are obtained from the manufacturers (Thermo-Fisher Incorporated, Headquarters at Waltham, MA USA 02451). These include—electrophoresis buffer, POP7 polymer and HiDi formamide. Formamide is stored in

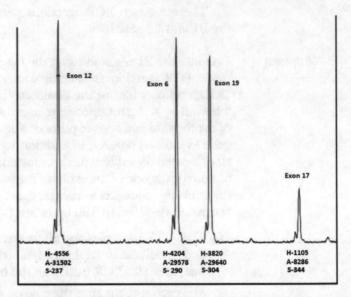

Fig. 1 A sample electropherogram generated by the Applied Biosystems' Gene Mapper Software. The figure shows the peaks corresponding to the PCR-amplified products of RB1 exons 12, 17, and 19 as displayed by Gene Mapper. The peak labeled as Exon 6 represents the internal control, which is exon 6 of the TGFB1 gene on chromosome 5. The height (H), area (A), and size (S) of each peak are given at the bottom

aliquots at −20 °C, and electrophoresis buffer and polymer for the ABI system are stored at 4 °C.

1. Take 2 μL of P2 reaction products; mix each with 10 μL HiDi formamide (Applied Biosystems Incorporated), and 0.5 μL of Liz size standard, in PCR tubes (0.2 mL) or into wells of a 96-well plate used with the ABI 3130 XL Genetic Analyzer system. For this step we use the Liz size standard, but any fluorescently labeled size standard compatible with the detection system of the genetic analyzer may be used.

2. Denature at 94 °C for 5 min, snap-chill on ice. Transfer the reactions from PCR tubes into a 96-well plate and load on to the ABI sequencer.

3. Detection and analysis of fragments is carried out with the Gene Mapper software.

4. In order to normalize the signal from each of the exons, you need to divide the signal from each exon peak by the signal from the internal control peak (Fig. 1). In addition, you need to include in each experiment the DNA samples from three normal control individuals, which are amplified similarly. Perform each PCR reaction in duplicate for patients' DNA and in triplicate for normal control DNA. The quantitative measure of the PCR products in each reaction is deduced from the peak areas for each exon obtained from the Gene Mapper software.

3.4 Determination of the Copy Number of Each Exon

1. Take the value of the peak areas of each exon of the test gene (in this case, *RB1*), and divide this by the peak area of the internal control, included in the same multiplex reaction (exon 5 of BIGH3). Determine peak area ratios for every exon of patients as well as normal controls.

2. Calculate the means and standard deviations of the ratios of peak areas obtained across duplicates/triplicates of each reaction. The mean peak area ratio of each exon from the test sample (Mt) is compared to the mean ratios obtained from three normal controls (Mc ± 2 SD). Use the value for normal controls from −2SD to +2SD as the range (*R*) for comparison with test values. If the value of Mt lies outside the range for controls by 20% or more, the sample is inferred to have a copy number change—either deletion or insertion, for Mt that is lower or higher than *R*, respectively (*see* **Note 5**).

4 Notes

1. Multiplexing of PCR reactions aids in reducing the total number of assays for large genes. For *RB1*, 27 exons were multiplexed into 10 reactions [6].

2. Combine primer sets into multiplex reactions. Primer combinations need to be tried and tested to get optimal conditions for multiplexing. Points to consider are similar annealing conditions of primers, difference in the sizes of PCR products so that each is clearly identifiable, and compatibility of different sets of primers to work in a multiplex reaction.

3. It is preferable to make a master mix of reagents that are common to all reactions and add the total volume of mix required to each reaction, to ensure more reproducible volumes. This will also reduce pipetting errors. Thus if ten reactions are being set up with the same set of primers and different DNA templates, calculate the volume of each of the above reagents (except DNA) needed for 11 reactions, and make up a master mix with those. Add the appropriate volume of master mix for each reaction. Then add template DNA individually.

4. Store fluorescently tagged primers away from light.

5. In principle, deletions or duplications of one allele should result in peak areas that are about 50% less or more respectively, than a normal control. However, we validated the method by testing DNA samples from retinoblastoma patients with known deletions and duplications, and found that the exon peak ratios varied from 20% to 50% lower or higher than the normal control values. These could reflect variable amplification efficiency for different templates. Hence, we apply 20% greater or lower than the normal range to interpret a copy number change.

References

1. Knudson AG Jr (1971) Mutation and cancer: statistical study of retinoblastoma. Proc Natl Acad Sci U S A 68:820–823

2. Richter SI, Vandezande K, Chen N et al (2003) Sensitive and efficient detection of RB1 gene mutations enhances care for families with retinoblastoma. Am J Hum Genet 72: 253–269

3. Xu K, Rosenwaks Z, Beaverson K et al (2004) Preimplantation genetic diagnosis for retinoblastoma: the first reported liveborn. Am J Ophthalmol 137:18–23

4. Valverde JR, Alonso J, Palacios I, Pestaña A (2005) RB1 gene mutation up-date, a meta-analysis based on 932 reported mutations available in a searchable database. BMC Genet 6:53

5. Price EA, Price K, Kolkiewicz K et al (2014) Spectrum of RB1 mutations identified in 403 retinoblastoma patients. J Med Genet 51:208–214

6. Parsam VL, Kannabiran C, Honavar S, Vemuganti GK, Ali MJ (2009) A comprehensive, sensitive and economical approach for detection of mutations in the RB1 gene in retinoblastoma. J Genet 88:517–527

7. Heath KE, Day IN, Humphries SE (2000) Universal primer quantitative fluorescent multiplex (UPQFM) PCR: a method to detect major and minor rearrangements of the low density lipoprotein receptor gene. J Med Genet 37:272–280

8. Sambrook J, Fritsch EF, Maniatis T (1989) Molecular cloning. A laboratory manual, 2nd edn. Cold Spring Harbor Laboratory Press, New York

Chapter 4

Using Methylation-Specific PCR to Study *RB1* Promoter Hypermethylation

Thaís M. McCormick and Maria Da Glória Da C. Carvalho

Abstract

It has increasingly been considered crucial the understanding of DNA methylation of Tumor Suppressor Gene (TSG) promoters, such as that of *retinoblastoma 1* gene (*RB1*), and its role during carcinogenesis. We present a detailed and optimized protocol of the methylation-specific PCR (MSP) technique to study *RB1* gene promoter hypermethylation.

Key words Methylation-specific PCR, Sodium bisulfite treatment, CpG island, *RB1*, Gene promoter methylation, 5-Methylcytosine, Tumor suppressor gene

1 Introduction

DNA methylation is an epigenetic regulatory mechanism consisting of the addition of a methyl radical in a cytosine followed by a guanine (CpG site) by enzymes called DNA methyltransferases (DNMTs) [1]. This process occurs in gene promoter regions in normal cells; however, the DNA methylation pattern in CpG islands is modified during carcinogenesis [2], wherein it is observed a global hypomethylation and a local hypermethylation, specially in TSGs promoters, such as *RB1*.

RB1 is a TSG encoding a nucleoprotein (pRb) involved in crucial steps of cell cycle [3]. The *RB1* gene silencing by aberrant methylation of the CpG island within its promoter region has been associated with a loss of pRb expression and progression of a number of cancer types [4, 5].

Faced with this background, it is clear that understanding of DNA methylation of TSG promoters, such as that of *RB1*, and its role during carcinogenesis deserves assessment by sensitive and reproducible techniques applicable to biological samples.

The current gold standard in the study of *RB1* promoter methylation pattern is the sodium bisulfite treatment, which can be used in different assays, such as methylation-specific PCR (MSP) [6].

Pedro G. Santiago-Cardona (ed.), *The Retinoblastoma Protein*, Methods in Molecular Biology, vol. 1726,
https://doi.org/10.1007/978-1-4939-7565-5_4, © Springer Science+Business Media, LLC 2018

Such a chemical procedure introduces methylation-dependent differences in a single-stranded DNA, as following: unmethylated cytosine residues are converted into uracil, under steps of (1) sulfonation of the cytosine by the addition of sodium bisulfite; (2) hydrolytic deamination to form a uracil-bisulfite derivative; and (3) alkali desulfonation to form a uracil. On the other hand, methylated cytosines (5-methylcytosine, 5-MeC) remain essentially nonreactive [7].

The sodium bisulfite treatment is highly single-stranded specific. Indeed, it is necessary a previous step to separate double stranded DNA, which is followed by the above mentioned chemical procedures that convert methylated cytosines into uracil, precipitation of treated genomic DNA (gDNA), and finally resuspension of the gDNA in water. This complete treatment is essentially performed in these four steps during at least 2 days.

After sodium bisulfite treatment, gDNA can undergo several assays in order to analyze the methylation profile of specific genes, such as direct sequencing, cloning followed by sequencing and Southern blotting analyses. However, MSP is a highly sensitive method to determine the methylation profile from 1 to 10 μg gDNA in 50 μg water, performed with lower time and costs.

MSP is a PCR protocol derivative, which is performed after the sodium bisulfite treatment and entails amplification of a gene of interest with primers specific for methylated and unmethylated DNA [6] (Fig. 1). Therefore, for each gene of interest, two primer pairs are necessary: one pair (sense and antisense) to amplify methylated DNA strands, and the other (sense and antisense) to amplify the unmethylated ones.

The design of specific primers is crucial to distinguish methylated from unmethylated DNA in bisulfite-modified DNA in a sensitive way, since the sequence differences resulting from bisulfite modification is essential to determine the required methylation profile. Therefore, if well performed, this technique can be useful to detect aberrant methylation pattern of a TSG in a neoplasia.

In what follows, a detailed protocol to study *RB1* promoter hypermethylation by MSP is presented.

2   Materials

2.1 Preparation of MSP Reaction Mix

1. 10× PCR Buffer Minus Mg^{2+}: 200 mM Tris-Cl (pH 8.4), 500 mM KCl.

2. 50 mM magnesium chloride.

3. dNTPs mix (25 mM each).

4. Primer mix (10 μM each).

5. 5 unit/μL *Taq* DNA Polymerase.

6. Autoclaved distilled water.

7. Bisulfite-modified gDNA.

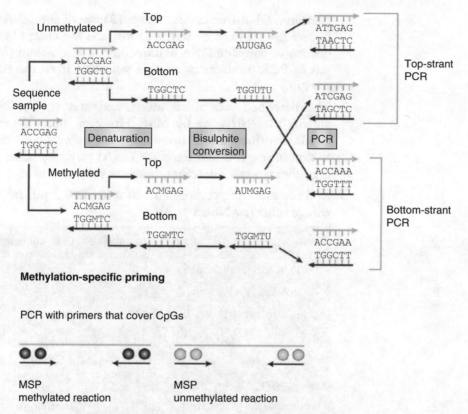

Methylation-specific priming

PCR with primers that cover CpGs

MSP
methylated reaction

MSP
unmethylated reaction

Fig. 1 Treatment of genomic DNA with sodium bisulfite followed by PCR amplification. This chemical treatment converts unmethylated cytosines to uracil residues, while methylated cytosine residues remain intact. As a consequence of such modification, the converted DNA is no longer self-complementary, and amplification of either the top or bottom DNA strand requires different primers. In MSP procedure, primers are methylation-specific. 5-methylcytosine residues are indicated in red Ms. *MSP* methylation-specific PCR. (Adapted from Laird, 2003 [8])

2.2 Methylation Specific PCR	1. 0.2 mL microcentrifuge tubes.
	2. Thermocycler.
	3. Mineral or silicone oil, optionally.

3 Methods

The cytosine sulfonation with sodium bisulfite step is a distinct procedure that the investigator needs to perform before the methylation specific PCR (MSP). The methods described below are focused exclusively on the methylation-specific PCR part of the technique.

3.1 Preparation of MSP Reaction Mix

1. As MSP is an effective technique capable of amplifying tiny amounts of DNA, appropriate precautions should be taken to avoid cross-contamination: (1) assemble amplification reac-

tions in a DNA-free environment; (2) use of aerosol-resistant barrier tips; (3) use of sterile gloves and lab coat; (4) use of primers or template DNA in individual reactions; and (5) analysis of PCR products in an area separated from the reaction assembly area.

2. The described procedure was tested and standardized to amplify the *RB1* gene by MSP. However, optimal reactions conditions (incubation times and temperatures, and concentration of reagents and template DNA) may vary when studying other targets. Therefore, trials are recommended.

3. Add the following components to a sterile 0.2 mL microcentrifuge tube: (*see* **Notes 1–3**):

Reagents	Volume (µL)	Final concentration
10× PCR buffer minus mg	5.0	1×
50 mM MgCl₂ (*see* **note 4**)	1.5	1.5 mM
Primers (10 µM each, *see* **note 5**)	2.0 each	0.4 µM each
dNTPs (25 mM each)	0.4	1.25 mM each
5 unit/µL *Taq* DNA polymerase	0.25	1.25 units
Autoclaved distilled water	34.85	Not applicable
Template DNA (3 µg/µL)	4.0	0.24 µg/µL

3.2 Methylation Specific PCR

1. After preparing the above mix including the template modified DNA in each tube, mix contents of the tubes and cover with 50 µL of mineral or silicone oil, if necessary (*see* **Note 6**).

2. Cap the tubes and centrifuge briefly to collect the contents.

3. Incubate the tubes in thermocycler and proceed with the following protocol:

Steps	Temperature (°C)	Time (min)
1. Initial DNA denaturation and polymerase activation (*see* **note 7**)	95	5
2. 35 cycles as follows:		
(a) Denaturation	95	1
(b) Annealing (*see* **note 8**)	60	1
(c) Extension	72	1
3. Final extension	72	10

4. Keep the MSP products at 4 °C until use.

5. Analyze the amplification products by polyacrylamide gel electrophoresis and visualize by silver nitrate staining. Use suitable molecular weight standards.

4 Notes

1. This reaction mix is prepared for a final volume of 50 μL, among which 4 μL is of gDNA. However, reaction size and concentrations may be altered to suit user preferences.

2. If desired, a master mix can be prepared for multiple reactions, to minimize reagent loss and to enable accurate pipetting.

3. The use of the reaction mix without template DNA as negative control is recommended.

4. Divalent cations, usually Mg^{2+}, are required for PCR reaction with thermostable DNA polymerases, such as *Taq* polymerase, since dNTPs and oligonucleotides bind Mg^{2+}. The routinely applied Mg^{2+} concentration is 1.5 mM, however increasing its concentration can be done depending on each combination of primers and template.

5. The amplification of a gene of interest, such as *RB1*, requires the preparation of two different MSP reaction mixes, each with a different primers pair: (1) forward and reverse primers for methylated DNA; and (2) forward and reverse primers for unmethylated DNA. Therefore, each reaction mix will have a total of 4.0 μL of primers: 2.0 μL for methylated plus 2.0 μL for unmethylated DNA. The specific primers for *RB1* suggested were described by Simpson et al. [5].

6. Mineral or silicone oil will prevent the evaporation of reaction mix, without compromising on MSP reaction quality. However, if the used thermocycler provides the option of heating the lid, the addition of such oil is not necessary.

7. *Taq* DNA polymerase is activated by a "hot start" at 94–95 °C. Such procedure increases sensitivity, specificity, and yield, thereby improving MSP results. Therefore, no modifications on this step are necessary.

8. The temperature of primers annealing to the template DNA is critical. The present annealing temperature was optimized to improve the yield of amplified DNA of interest by avoiding occurrence of nonspecific segments amplification and of primer dimers. Nevertheless, it is best to optimize the annealing conditions for each primer pair before first trial.

References

1. Muhonen P, Holthofer H (2008) Epigenetic and microRNA-mediated regulation in diabetes. Nephrol Dial Transplant 24:1088–1096. https://doi.org/10.1093/ndt/gfn728

2. Jaenisch R, Bird A (2003) Epigenetic regulation of gene expression: how the genome integrates intrinsic and environmental signals. Nat Genet 33(Suppl):245–254. https://doi.org/10.1038/ng1089

3. Lee W-H, Shew J-Y, Hong FD et al (1987) The retinoblastoma susceptibility gene encodes a nuclear phosphoprotein associated with DNA binding activity. Nature 329:642–645. https://doi.org/10.1038/329642a0

4. McCormick TM, Canedo NH, Furtado YL et al (2015) Association between human papillomavirus and Epstein-Barr virus DNA and gene promoter methylation of RB1 and CDH1 in the cervical lesions: a transversal study. Diagn Pathol 10:59. https://doi.org/10.1186/s13000-015-0283-3

5. Simpson DJ, Hibberts NA, McNicol AM et al (2000) Loss of pRb expression in pituitary adenomas is associated with methylation of the RB1 CpG island. Cancer Res 60:1211–1216

6. Herman JG, Graff JR, Myöhänen S et al (1996) Methylation-specific PCR: a novel PCR assay for methylation status of CpG islands. Proc Natl Acad Sci U S A 93:9821–9826

7. Clark SJ, Harrison J, Paul CL, Frommer M (1994) High sensitivity mapping of methylated cytosines. Nucleic Acids Res 22:2990–2997

8. Laird PW (2003) Early detection: the power and the promise of DNA methylation markers. Nat Rev Cancer 3:253–266. https://doi.org/10.1038/nrc1045

Chapter 5

Detection of Aberrant DNA Methylation Patterns in the *RB1* Gene

Sumadi Lukman Anwar and Ulrich Lehmann

Abstract

The retinoblastoma protein (pRb) plays a central role in the regulation of cell cycle by interaction with members of the E2F transcription factor family. As a tumor suppressor protein, pRb is frequently dysregulated in several major cancers. In addition to mutations, inactivation of pRb is also caused by epigenetic mechanisms including alterations of DNA methylation. There are three CpG islands located within the *RB1* gene that encodes pRb that are closely associated with the regulation of pRb expression. Aberrant DNA methylation at the *RB1* gene has been reported in sporadic retinoblastoma as well as other cancers including glioblastoma, hepatocellular carcinoma, and breast cancer. Recent studies have revealed that the *RB1* gene is imprinted. Therefore, quantitative analysis is required to detect aberrations in DNA methylation associated with imprint deregulation. Pyrosequencing® is considered as the method of choice for quantitative and reproducible analysis of DNA methylation with single base resolution. In this chapter, we provide a detailed protocol for the quantitative analysis of *RB1* gene methylation using bisulfite Pyrosequencing®.

Key words *RB1* gene, DNA methylation, Quantitative, Imprinting, Bisulfite pyrosequencing

1 Introduction

The retinoblastoma tumor suppressor gene (*RB1*) has emerged as a focus of cancer research during the past 30 years after its discovery [1, 2]. The *RB1* gene is the first identified human tumor suppressor gene and is often inactivated in different types of cancer [2]. Germline mutations of the *RB1* gene confer patients with high risk of childhood onset retinoblastoma [3]. The retinoblastoma protein (pRb) plays a central role in cell cycle regulation through interaction with E2F transcription factors [2, 4]. The unphosphorylated state as an active form of pRb is able to bind and inhibit E2F transcription factors resulting in cell cycle arrest in the G1 phase. On the other hand, phosphorylation of pRb through cyclin-dependent kinases (CDKs) causes release of E2F proteins from the pRb-E2F complex resulting in transcriptional activation and cell cycle progression. In addition, pRb regulates several important biological

Pedro G. Santiago-Cardona (ed.), *The Retinoblastoma Protein*, Methods in Molecular Biology, vol. 1726,
https://doi.org/10.1007/978-1-4939-7565-5_5, © Springer Science+Business Media, LLC 2018

pathways including cell differentiation, cell survival, DNA damage responses, and senescence [2, 4].

The *RB1* tumor suppressor gene is often inactivated in cancer. Possible mechanisms responsible for inactivation are mutations, loss of heterozygosity (LOH), chromosomal rearrangements, and epigenetic reprograming [2, 5]. Inactivation of *RB1* gene is generally caused by a combination of genetic and epigenetic alterations of the two alleles; in fact, that tumor suppressor genes require two hits for their inactivation has been first described for the *RB1* gene [6, 7]. Aberrant DNA methylation of gene regulatory elements is the most common epigenetic mechanism causing loss of gene expression [8]. In mammals, DNA methylation takes place only at the base cytosine if it is followed by guanine. The CpG dinucleotide is unevenly distributed in the human genome [9]. Genomic regions densely populated by CpG dinucleotides are called CpG islands and those located near the transcriptional start sites play a major role as regulatory element for transcription. The methylation status of CpG islands located at the promoter region is associated with transcriptional silencing and delayed replication during mitosis. Most CpGs are methylated except those located near active gene promoters [10, 11]. Approximately 60–70% of gene promoters are associated with one or more CpG islands, which function as regulatory elements of gene promoters. CpG dinucleotides outside of promoter regions are usually methylated. DNA methylation plays a vital role in diverse biological processes, like regulation of cellular differentiation, embryonic development, X-chromosome inactivation, genomic imprinting, and allele-specific expression [9–11].

The human *RB1* gene is located at chromosome 13q14 (USCS Genome Browser h19, chr13:48,877,883–48,937,093) [1, 3]. There are three CpG islands located within the human *RB1* locus (Fig. 1) [12]. A 1042 bp CpG island with a total of 106 CpG dinucleotides is located in the 5′ region of the gene (UCSC Genome Browser h19, chr13:48,877,460–48,878,501) and contains the basal promoter of the *RB1* gene [12, 13]. This CpG island remains unmethylated during embryonic development as well as in adult healthy tissues. Hypermethylation of the CpG island located at the *RB1* promoter has been shown and is associated with diminished pRb protein expression [13]. Hypermethylation of the *RB1* gene has been reported in retinoblastoma, glioblastoma, breast cancer, and bladder cancer [2]. The second CpG island (UCSC Genome Browser h19, chr13:48,890,958–48,891,549) is located in intron 2 with a total of 42 CpG dinucleotides. However, the second CpG island is commonly methylated across different tissues suggesting lack of regulatory function. The third CpG island is also located in intron 2 just upstream of exon 3. It spans 1222 bp with 85 CpG dinucleotides altogether (UCSC Genome browser h19,

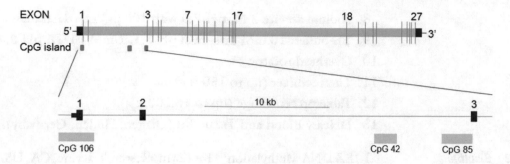

Fig. 1 Structure of *RB1* gene and location of the CpG islands. The *RB1* gene is located at chromosome 13q14 with 27 exons and 3 identified CpG islands. The first CpG islands (CpG106) are located at the regulatory promoter region and the second (CpG42) and the third (CpG85) CpG islands are located at the intron 2

chr13:48,892,636–48,893,857) [12]. Recent studies have revealed that the *RB1* gene is indeed imprinted [14]. Genomic imprinting is a specific epigenetic mechanism leading to parent-of-origin specific gene expression [15]. Imprinting is mainly established by differential DNA methylation as well as histone modification [16]. The regulatory elements for the establishment of imprinting processes are known as differentially methylated regions (DMR). If the DMR regulates more than one gene, the regulatory region is called an imprinting control region (ICR) [16, 17]. The DMR and ICR show allele specific DNA methylation. For the human *RB1* imprinting, the DMR is located at the third CpG island in intron 2 just upstream of exon 3 (known as "CpG85"). This DMR originated from the *KIAA0649* gene on chromosome 9 through retro-transposition. In the human genome, this *RB1*-DMR is exclusively methylated at the maternal allele whereas in mouse, the *Rb1* gene is not imprinted. Differential methylation of the *RB1*-DMR regulates expression of the alternative transcript E2B. The E2B transcript functions as a long non-coding RNA that can inhibit the expression of the main RB1 transcript [14].

2   Materials

2.1   DNA Extraction

1. Ethanol 70% and absolute.
2. Proteinase K.
3. Proteinase-K buffer: 50 mM Tris–HCl pH 8.1, 1 mM EDTA pH 8.0, and 0.5% Tween 20.
4. Phenol–chloroform–isoamyl alcohol (in a 25:24:1 ratio).
5. Chloroform.
6. Isopropanol.
7. RNase A.

8. Sodium acetate 3 M, pH 7.0 with 100 µg/mL dextran.

9. TE-buffer: 10 mM Tris–HCl pH 8.1, 1 mM EDTA pH 8.0.

10. Overhead rotator.

11. Thermomixer (up to $150 \times g$).

12. Tabletop centrifuge (up to $16,200 \times g$).

13. DNeasy Blood and Tissue Kit (Qiagen, Hilden, Germany).

2.2 Bisulfite Conversion

1. EZ DNA Methylation™ Kit (ZymoResearch, Irvine, CA, USA).

2. Ethanol.

3. Tabletop centrifuge (up to $16,200 \times g$).

4. Heating block with cover (to provide light protection and even heating).

2.3 Polymerase Chain Reaction (PCR)

1. Taq-Polymerase (Platinum Taq® DNA polymerase, Thermo-Fisher Scientific) including PCR buffer and $MgCl_2$.

2. dNTPs.

3. *RB1* primer sets (100 µM): for the PCR-based amplification of CpG islands located at the *RB1* gene from bisulfite-converted DNA and sequencing primer (*see* example of primers at Table 1).

4. PCR tubes or plates.

5. Thermocycler.

2.4 Pyrosequencing

1. Pyrosequencing system (Qiagen, Hilden, Germany).

2. Pyro Q-CpG™ software (Qiagen).

3. Reagent cartridges (Qiagen).

4. Capillary cartridges (Qiagen).

5. Dispensing unit/Cartridge holder (Qiagen).

6. Pyrosequencing reagent kit (Qiagen, Hilden, Germany).

7. Primers for sequencing reaction.

8. Biotinylated PCR products.

9. Streptavidin Sepharose® HP (GE Healthcare, Chalfont StGiles, GB).

10. PCR plates (96-well plate for PyroMark® Q96 ID system).

11. Plate mixer (100 up to $200 \times g$).

12. Pyrosequencing plates (PyroMark Q96 Plate Low).

13. Vacuum workstation with the appropriate filter tips and troughs (Qiagen).

14. PyroMark™ Binding buffer (Qiagen).

15. Denaturation solution: 0.2 N NaOH.

Table 1
Examples of primers for bisulfite Pyrosequencing® assays for the *RB1* gene

Primer	Forward	Reverse	*T* (°C)	MgCl$_2$	Sequencing
CpG106	GGGGGTGGTTTTGGGTAGAAG	Tail-AAACCRAACRCRCCCTCCCC	65	2.5	TGGTTTTGGGTAGAAGTA
CpG42	GGGTTTAGATTTTTATTGTTGAG	Tail-CRACCAAAACCAAAACACCT	60	2.5	AGATTTTATTGTTGAGTTG
CpG85	GGTAGGGTAGTTTTGGAAATGTTTAAG	Tail-AACCACAAACCCTTACCC	60	1.5	AGTTTTGGAAATGTTTAAGAT

16. Washing buffer concentrate (Qiagen, Hilden, Germany).

17. Annealing buffer (Qiagen, Hilden, Germany).

18. High purity water.

19. Ethanol.

20. Heating block (heating up to 80 °C) suitable for 96-wells plate for PyroMark Q96.

21. Sample Prep Thermoplate Low (Qiagen).

22. PSQ Assay design software.

23. Sequence Conversion Tool.

3 Methods

3.1 Assay Design

After bisulfite treatment both strands are no longer complementary. Therefore, to design primers for DNA methylation analysis there are principally four possibilities: the sense or antisense strand and both in forward or reverse orientation. For designing Pyrosequencing® assays, Biotage® has developed the PSQ Assay design software. The DNA sequence obtained after in silico bisulfite treatment can be copied directly into the program (online software for bisulfite conversion sequence, *see* **Note 1**). Afterwards one has to indicate the region that will be amplified and sequenced. Manual modification of primer position and length is possible considering melting temperature, possible secondary structures within the template, and primer dimer formation. There are also available free online software tools to develop Pyrosequencing® assays (*see* **Note 2**). After bisulfite conversion, the DNA sequence changes dramatically with turning all C outside a CpG dinucleotide into T resulting in challenges for PCR primer design due to reduced sequence complexity. To develop optimized primers for DNA methylation analysis using Pyrosequencing®, one should avoid CpG sites within primer binding sites (especially the first five nucleotides at the 3′ region known as seed sequence). If CpG sites are included within the primer-binding site (supposed to be outside the seed sequence), the primer has to contain a wobble site at this position, i.e., Y (for C/T) for forward direction and R (for G/A) for reverse direction. SNPs and other genomic variations with the selected primer binding sites should be avoided to minimize potential bias of the amplification and sequencing reaction. Ideally primers should contain a minimum of four converted cytosines to increase specificity for fully bisulfite converted DNA. General rules for primer design including GC content should not be more than 60%, annealing temperature should 55–65 °C, avoiding repetitive sequences and homopolymers are warranted. For bisulfite pyrosequencing, primers used for PCR are also recommended to use universal biotinylated primer and addition of a universal tail either at the forward or the reverse primer (*see* **Note 3**) [18]. The length of PCR products should be no longer than 350 bp to avoid secondary structures of the single stranded template in the sequencing reaction, which takes place at 28 °C (*see* below). For samples from FFPE tissues, the amplicon should be no longer than 150 bp because of the formalin-induced DNA fragmentation. One should add always at least one conversion control (dispensation of C for a position where a C has been converted to T or, for the reverse strand, dispensation of G) in order to control for completeness of the bisulfite treatment (*see* **Note 4**). A sample assay design for *RB1* CpG promoter island 106 is shown in Fig. 2.

3.2 DNA Extraction (For Fresh-Frozen Specimens)

1. Resuspend 10–30 g of fresh-frozen tissues in 750 μL Proteinase K-buffer and 25 μL Proteinase K.

2. Incubate in a thermo-shaker at 55 °C and 50 × *g* overnight.

3. Add 750 μL phenol–chloroform–isoamyl alcohol and mix by inverting for 30 min.

4. Centrifuge at room temperature for 10 min at 16,200 × *g*. The mixture will be separated into three layers.

5. Take the aqueous phase and repeat **steps 3** and **4** until no interphase is visible any more.

RB1 promoter (CpG 106)

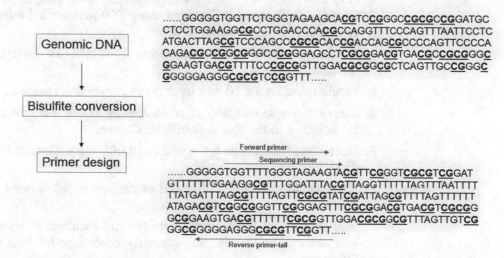

Fig. 2 Assay design for pyrosequencing run. To design primers for PCR and sequencing, we need to convert genomic DNA sequence by replacing independent cytosines into thymines (use online software for bisulfite conversion sequence). Primers are designed complementary to the converted sequence following the general rules (*see* Subheading 3)

6. Add 50 µg RNase A and incubate in a thermo-shaker for 30 min at 37 °C and 80 × g.

7. Repeat **steps 3** and **4**, to remove the RNase A.

8. Add 750 µL chloroform to the aqueous phase, mix by inverting 30 min.

9. Subsequently centrifuge for 3 min, 16,200 × g at room temperature.

10. Precipitate the DNA by adding 0.1 volumes of 3 M sodium acetate (pH 7.0)/100 µg/mL dextran and 2.5 volumes 100% ethanol and inversion of the solution.

11. Wash the precipitate with 500 µL of 70% ethanol and dissolve it in 500 µL TE buffer.

12. DNA extraction using a commercial kit from Qiagen (QIAamp DNA micro kit) and other commercial companies also performs well for bisulfite pyrosequencing.

13. The extracted DNA should be quantified using spectrophotometer to determine the concentration and general quality.

3.3 Bisulfite Treatment

1. For bisulfite conversion, we normally use the EZ DNA Methylation™ Kit (Zymo Research) and perform bisulfite treatment according to the manufacturer's protocol (*see* **Note 5**).

2. For optimum bisulfite conversion, 1 µg genomic DNA is mixed with 5 µL M-Dilution Buffer and distilled water to reach a total volume of 50 µL and then incubated at 42 °C for 15 min.

3. Add 100 µL of CT Conversion Reagent to each sample (CT Conversion Reagent is dissolved using 750 µL distilled water and 210 µL M-Dilution buffer).

4. Incubate at 50 °C in a thermo-shaker overnight (12–16 h) in the dark.

5. Incubate on ice for 10 min to stop the conversion reaction.

6. Mix each sample with 400 µL of M-Binding Buffer and transfer the solution to the Zymo-Spin™ IC Column.

7. Centrifuge for 30 s at full speed (>10,000 × g). Discard the flow-through.

8. Add 100 µL M-Wash Buffer and centrifuge at full speed for 30 s.

9. Add 200 µL M-Desulfonation Buffer and incubate at room temperature for 15 min. Subsequently, centrifuge for 30 s at full speed.

10. Add 200 µL M-Wash Buffer, centrifuge at full speed for 30 s and repeat this step one more time.

11. Place the column into a 1.5 mL microcentrifuge tube.

12. Elute the converted DNA by adding about 40 μL of M-Elution Buffer directly to the column matrix and centrifugation at full speed for 30 s (*see* **Note 6**).

3.4 PCR Amplification of Bisulfite-Converted DNA

1. PCR reactions for amplification of bisulfite converted DNA for subsequent Pyrosequencing® analysis are performed using 0.4 μM non-tailed, 0.4 μM universal biotinylated, and 0.04 μM tailed primer, 10 ng bisulfite treated DNA, 0.2 mM dNTP, 0.02 unit/ μL Taq polymerase (*see* **Note 7**), PCR buffer, and water to add the total volume of 25 μL. Please *see* Table 1 for examples of primers used for *RB1* gene DNA methylation analysis.

2. The optimal PCR reaction has also to be determined for each primer set by adjusting $MgCl_2$ concentration (usually 1.5 or 2.5 mM) and the annealing temperature.

3. The PCR should be performed using the following thermo-cycling conditions: 15 min at 95 °C; 45–60 cycles of (94 °C for 30 s; annealing temperature (*see* Table 1) for 30 s; 72 °C for 30 s); 72 °C for 5 min (*see* **Note 8**).

4. Specificity and amount of PCR amplicons should be verified using gel electrophoresis (4% acrylamide) under electric field 100 V for 30 min to visualize clear and distinct band without unspecific byproducts.

3.5 Bisulfite Pyrosequencing®

3.5.1 Sample Preparation

1. Switch on heating block (80 ° C).

2. Switch on the PyroMark Q96MD system to allow 90 min warm-up for stabilization of the CCD camera before initial capture.

3. Open the PyroQ-CpG software and create the plate set up by dragging the assay designs into the working plate. Press "Tool and -> Volume Information" and the system will automatically calculate amount of enzyme, substrate, and nucleotides (A, C, G, T) that are required to be loaded to the individual cartridges.

4. Fill the Vacuum Prepstation with the corresponding buffers (~180 mL of 70% ethanol, Denaturation Solution 0.2 N NaOH, Wash Buffer, and Milli-Q grade water).

5. Prepare the PyroMark Binding Buffer mixture as follows: 47 μL PyroMark Binding Buffer, 3 μL streptavidin Sepharose® beads, 20 μL dH_2O.

6. Dispense 70 μL of Binding Buffer mixture into each well of a 96-well plate and add 10 μL of PCR product.

7. After sealing the plate with an adhesive cover, incubate the plate for 5 min with vigorous shaking at $150 \times g$.

8. Prepare the Annealing Buffer mixture as follows: 11 µL PyroMark annealing buffer, 1 µL sequencing primer (0.83 µM concentration).

9. Dispense 12 µL of Annealing Buffer mixture into a PyroMark Q96 HS Plate.

3.5.2 Strand Separation

1. Switch on vacuum, apply to the vacuum workstation and wash filter tips with Milli-Q water for approximately 10 s.

2. Lower the filter tips into the 96-well PCR plate containing bead and the immobilized PCR templates on to capture them into the filter tips.

3. Carefully take out the aspiration device from the plate (beware not to lose the beads containing PCR DNA fragments on top of the filter tips).

4. Wash beads by placing the vacuum prep tool into 70% ethanol and let the solution flush through the filters for 5 s.

5. Denature the double stranded DNAs by placing the vacuum prep tool into the Denaturation Solution and flushing it through the filters for 10 s.

6. Wash the bead once again with the Wash Buffer by flushing it through the filters for 5 s.

7. Remove all residual liquids from the beads by rising and tilting the aspiration device while vacuum is still on for 5 s.

8. Switch off the vacuum using the switch on-off panel at the vacuum prep tool handle and wait until the pressure is back to zero (*see* **Note 9**).

9. Release the beads in a PyroMark Q96 HS Plate filled with the mixture of annealing buffer and sequencing primer by gently shaking the vacuum prep tool for 30 s (vacuum off, of course).

10. Seal the PyroMark Q96 HS Plate with an adhesive cover.

3.5.3 Primer Annealing

1. Place the PyroMark Q96 HS Plate at the preheated heating block (80 °C) for 2 min and cover it with the thermoplate to reduce evaporation within the wells.

2. Remove the plate from the heating block and leave the samples on the bench for 10 min in order to cool down to room temperature.

3.5.4 Pyrosequencing®
Reaction

1. Prior to loading the nucleotides into the individual cartridges, centrifuge for 5 min 13,000 × *g* at 4 °C to sediment any kind of particles to avoid their transfer into the cartridges (*see* **Note 10**).

2. As documented at the "Volume Information" as stated at the **step 3**, fill the required amount of enzyme, substrate, and nucleotides into each individual cartridge.

3. Place the cartridges into the cartridge holder, place the cartridge as well as the Pyrosequencing® plate into the PyroMark Q96MD, and close the lid.

4. After performing the dispensation test, run the assay within the Pyro Q-CpG software. Once the run is finished, data can be extracted.

3.6 Pyrogram Evaluation

The outcome of the Pyrosequencing® run is displayed in a graph called Pyrogram (Fig. 3). DNA methylation levels are shown as signal intensities (arbitrary units, a.u.) highlighted usually in gray. The percentage of DNA methylation values (on top of the gray boxes) refers to average methylation level for the respective CpG site within the assay. A conversion control (at least on, preferably more) should also be included during assay design as a quality control for completeness of bisulfite treatment. Default settings of the Pyro Q-CpG software set background thresholds of 7.0% for conversion controls (yellow colored) and 4.5% for CpG sites, that can be adjusted (Qiagen recommends percentages of 9.5 and 6.5, respectively). The signal intensity of each peak should be distinct from the background signals and the peak height of a single nucleotide incorporation should be above 30–50 a.u. At least two Pyrosequencing® runs for each measurement should be performed to obtain reliable data. Decreased peak heights, especially found in long assays with more than 80–100 nucleotides, indicate declining

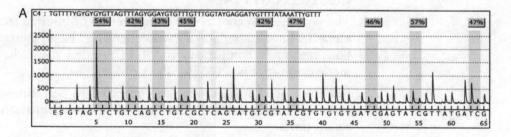

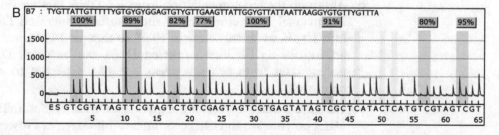

Fig. 3 Pyrogram of multiple CpG sites within CpG106, CpG42, and CpG85 of the *RB1* gene. The Y-axis denotes DNA methylation intensity (in a.u.; arbitrary units) and the X-axis is the nucleotide dispensation order. DNA methylation of several CpG sites (highlighted in gray) is quantified in a single Pyrosequencing run. The percentage DNA methylation levels of each CpG site are shown at the top of gray highlight. Conversion controls are shown as yellow bar

enzyme activity. Therefore, it is recommended under most circumstances to develop assays less than 100 nucleotides in length to produce high quality pyrograms.

4   Notes

1. Primers for bisulfite PCR are designed based on genomic DNA after bisulfite conversion. One can decide which DNA strands will be converted either sense or antisense, therefore one has four possibilities in designing primers for bisulfite PCR. To generate the DNA sequence after bisulfite conversion, one can use the following online software: http://biq-analyzer.bioinf.mpi-inf.mpg.de/tools/BiConverter/index.php

2. Online software that can be used for designing primers for bisulfite methylation PCR: MethPrimer (http://www.uro-gene.org/methprimer/), and MethylPrimer Express (http://www.appliedbiosystems.com/absite/us/en/home/support/software-community/freeab-software.html).

3. For bisulfite Pyrosequencing®, it is recommended for the PCR to use one primer with tail (either forward or reverse primer) and an additional universal biotinylated primer. The sequence for the tail primer is GGGACACCGCTGATCGTTTA followed by the sequence of forward or reverse primer. The sequence for the universal biotinylated primer is GGGACACCGCTGATCGTTTA.

4. The possibility to control the completeness of bisulfite treatment is a huge advantage of Pyrosequencing®-based methylation analysis in comparison to all PCR-based methods, as methylation-specific PCR (MSP) or qMSP.

5. Kits from other suppliers are also expected to perform well. However, we did not perform a comprehensive comparison in recent times.

6. Although the recommendation from EZ DNA Methylation™ Kit manual is to elute finally the bisulfite converted DNA into 10 µL, we usually elute in 40 µL so that per PCR reaction, around 25 ng bisulfite-converted DNA can be used. DNA polymerases from other vendors are also expected to perform well.

7. We have extensive yearlong experiences with PlatiniumTaq® DNA polymerase and can recommend this enzyme. However, we didn't perform a comprehensive comparison of different polymerases from different vendors. Therefore, other Taq Polymerases might work as well.

8. The final extension step really improves the performance of the pyrosequencing results.

9. If you put the filter tips of the vacuum devise too early into the pyrosequencing plate with annealing buffer and pyrosequencing primer ("too early" means: when there is still some negative pressure), the reaction mixture will be sucked away and will thereby be lost irreversibly.

10. The needles through which enzyme, substrate, and the nucleotides are dispensed are so narrow, that even very tiny pieces of dust can cause complete clogging. Therefore, it is very important to pipette are "clean" solution without any remaining particles.

References

1. Friend SH, Bernards RA, Rogelj S, Weinberg RA, Rapaport JM, Albert DM, Dryja TP (1986) A human DNA segment with properties of the gene that predisposes to retinoblastoma and osteosarcoma. Nature 323(6089):643–646

2. Benavente CA, Dyer DA (2015) Genetics and epigenetics of human retinoblastoma. Annu Rev Pathol 10:547–562

3. Lohmann DR (1999) RB1 gene mutations in retinoblastoma. Hum Mutat 14(4):283–288

4. Harbour JW, Dean DC (2000) Rb function in cell-cycle regulation and apoptosis. Nat Cell Biol 2(4):65–67

5. Di Fiore R, D'Anneo A, Tesoriere G, Vento R (2013) RB1 in cancer: different mechanisms of RB1 inactivation and alterations of pRb pathway in tumorigenesis. J Cell Physiol 228:1676–1687

6. Knudson AG (1971) Mutation and cancer: statistical study of retinoblastoma. Proc Natl Acad Sci U S A 68(4):820–823

7. Knudson AG (2001) Two genetic hits (more or less) to cancer. Nat Rev Cancer 1(2):157–162

8. Deaton AM, Bird A (2011) CpG islands and the regulation of transcription. Genes Dev 25(10):1010–1022

9. Ziller MJ, Gu H, Müller F, Donaghey J, Tsai LT-Y, Kohlbacher O, De Jager PL, Rosen ED, Bennett D, Bernstein BE, Gnirke A, Meissner A (2013) Charting a dynamic DNA methylation landscape of the human genome. Nature 500(7463):477–481

10. Antequera F, Bird A (1993) Number of CpG islands and genes in human and mouse. Proc Natl Acad Sci U S A 90(24):11995–11999

11. Robertson KD (2005) DNA methylation and human disease. Nat Rev Genet 6(8):597–610

12. Anwar SL, Krech T, Hasemeier B, Schipper E, Schweitzer N, Vogel A, Kreipe H, Lehmann U (2014) Deregulation of RB1 expression by loss of imprinting in human hepatocellular carcinoma. J Pathol 233(4):392–401

13. Gonzalez-Gomez P, Bello MJ, Alonso ME, Arjona D, Lomas J, Campos JM, Isla A, Rey JA (2003) CpG island methylation status and mutation analysis of the RB1 gene essential promoter region and protein-binding pocket domain in nervous system tumours. Br J Cancer 88(1):109–114

14. Kanber D, Berulava T, Ammerpohl O, Mitter D, Richter J, Siebert R, Horsthemke B, Lohmann D, Buiting K (2009) The human retinoblastoma gene is imprinted. PLoS Genet 5(12):1–9

15. Horsthemke B (2014) In brief: genomic imprinting and imprinting diseases. J Pathol 232(5):485–487

16. Ferguson-Smith AC (2011) Genomic imprinting: the emergence of an epigenetic paradigm. Nat Rev Genet 12(8):565–575

17. Barlow DP (2011) Genomic imprinting: a mammalian epigenetic discovery model. Annu Rev Genet 45:379–403

18. Royo JL, Hidalgo M, Ruiz A (2007) Pyrosequencing protocol using a universal biotinylated primer for mutation detection and SNP genotyping. Nat Protoc 2(7):1734–1739

Chapter 6

Detection of Retinoblastoma Protein Phosphorylation by Immunoblot Analysis

Pedro G. Santiago-Cardona, Jaileene Pérez-Morales, and Jonathan González-Flores

Abstract

The retinoblastoma tumor suppressor protein (pRb) is a preeminent tumor suppressor that acts as a cell cycle repressor, specifically as an inhibitor of the G1–S transition of the cell cycle. pRb is a phosphoprotein whose function is repressed by extensive phosphorylation in several key residues, and therefore, pRb's phosphorylation status has become a surrogate for pRb activity. In particular, hyperphosphorylation of pRb has been associated with pathological states such as cancer, and therefore, assessing pRb's phosphorylation status is increasingly gaining diagnostic and prognostic value, may be used to inform therapeutic decisions, and is also an important tool for the cancer biologists seeking an understanding of the molecular etiology of cancer. In this chapter, we discuss an immunoblot protocol to detect pRb phosphorylation in two residues, serine 612 and threonine 821, in protein extracts from cancer cells.

Key words Retinoblastoma protein, Immunoblot, Phosphorylation, Cell cycle control, Oncogenesis, Lung adenocarcinoma

1 Introduction

The retinoblastoma tumor suppressor protein (pRb) is a preeminent tumor suppressor that acts as a cell cycle repressor, specifically as an inhibitor of the G1–S transition of the cell cycle [1, 2]. Given pRb's role as a cell cycle repressor, it is expected that pRb function is impaired in most human cancers. A mechanism of loss of pRb function may be genetic mutations in the *RB1* locus encoding the pRb protein. However, this mechanism of pRb inactivation is seen only in a small subset of human cancers, primordially in small cell lung carcinomas, osteosarcomas, and in retinoblastomas [3]. Instead, the vast majority of human tumors experience loss of pRb function via a physiologically common mechanism of pRb inactivation consisting on pRb hyperphosphorylation by Cyclin-dependent kinases (Cdks) [4]. It is a common occurrence in human cancers to have overactivated Cdks, either by the genetic amplification of the

Pedro G. Santiago-Cardona (ed.), *The Retinoblastoma Protein*, Methods in Molecular Biology, vol. 1726, https://doi.org/10.1007/978-1-4939-7565-5_6, © Springer Science+Business Media, LLC 2018

genes coding for them or for their cyclin activating subunits, or by the repression of the activity of Cdk inhibitors [4]. Therefore, in a cancer context, pRb is usually hyperphosphorylated and consequently impaired from its cell cycle repressive function.

pRb's phosphorylation state has become a surrogate for pRb function, pRb hyperphosphorylation strongly indicating functional inactivation. Particularly telling about pRb function is the phosphorylation of serine and threonine residues in pRb's central pocket domain and its C-terminal. These phosphorylations are particularly disruptive of pRb's function as a cell cycle repressor, since they disrupt pRb's interaction with members of the E2F transcription factor family, an interaction that is central for pRb's tumor suppressive role [1, 2]. pRb phosphorylation in the pocket and C-terminal domains is mechanistically associated with overproliferation and with the molecular etiology of cancer [5–7]. Therefore, assessing pRb's phosphorylation state, specially phosphorylations occurring in the pocket and C-terminal domains, has become extremely informative regarding the oncogenic proclivity of a cell, and, when conducted in human tumor samples, it can provide valuable diagnostic, prognostic, and therapy responsiveness information.

In this chapter, we describe a procedure for detecting hyperphosphorylation in two key pRb residues mediating its function as a cell cycle repressor, namely, phosphorylation of serine 612 (in the pocket domain), and of threonine 821 (C-terminal). These two phosphorylations have been mechanistically proven to strongly affect pRb-E2F interactions and are therefore strongly implicated in abrogating pRb's tumor suppressive capacity as well as in oncogenicity [5, 8–12]. This protocol describes the detection of such phosphorylations by immunoblot analysis using protein extracts from lung cancer cell lines. Therefore, this protocol will definitively be of great value for molecular cancer biologists seeking to pursue in vitro studies of the molecular aspects associated to the loss of cell cycle control commonly observed in human cancers.

2   Materials

Prepare all solutions using distilled water and analytical grade reagents. Unless otherwise noted, the reagents and solutions below can be stored at room temperature. Follow all waste disposal regulations when disposing of waste materials.

2.1 Cell Lysis and Protein Extraction

1. 1× Phosphate-Buffered Saline (PBS). For convenience, many vendors provide premade PBS either in the form of a solution, or as premixed components ready to be diluted in water. If these are not available, the standard recipe for 1× PBS should work well. To prepare 1× PBS, dissolve 8 g NaCl, 0.2 g KCl,

1.44 g $Na_2HPO_4 \cdot 2\,H_2O$, and 0.24 g of KH_2PO_4 in 800 ml of water. Adjust the pH to 7.2 with HCL, and add distilled water to complete the volume to 1 l.

2. Cell scrapers or Trypsin–EDTA solution (*see* **Note 1**).

3. RIPA buffer. For convenience, we use the premixed 10× RIPA buffer from Cell Signaling (Cat. No. 9806). However, the standard recipe can also be used, which consists of 10 mM Tris–HCl, pH 8.0, 1 mM EDTA, 0.5 mM EGTA, 1% (v/v) NP-40 (or 1% Triton X-100, if NP-40 is not available), 0.5% (v/v) sodium deoxycholate, 0.1% (v/v) SDS, and 150 mM NaCl.

4. Protease and phosphatase inhibitor cocktails, use according to manufacturer's specifications (*see* **Note 2**).

2.2 SDS Polyacrylamide Gel Electrophoresis

1. 1.5 M Tris–HCl, pH 8.8. To prepare, dissolve 181.7 g of Tris base in 800 ml H_2O. Adjust pH to 8.8 with concentrated HCl (*see* **Note 3**). Add H_2O to complete the volume to 1 l. Store at 4 °C.

2. 0.5 M Tris–HCl, pH 6.8. To prepare, dissolve 60.6 g of Tris base in 800 ml H_2O. Adjust pH to 6.8 with concentrated HCl. Add H_2O to complete the volume to 1 l. Store at 4 °C (*see* **Note 4**).

3. 30% acrylamide–Bis-acrylamide solution (*see* **Note 5**). Please be aware that polyacrylamide is toxic. Carefully read the accompanying Materials Safety Data Sheet for specific instructions on how to handle and dispose polyacrylamide solutions.

4. Ammonium persulfate (APS): 10% (w/v) APS solution in water. Dissolve 0.5 g ammonium persulfate in 5 ml of dH_2O, make aliquots and store at −20 °C. Avoid repeated freezing and thawing cycles. It is recommended that the aliquots are of a small amount. Avoid reusing left overs.

5. Tetramethylethylenediamine (TEMED).

6. 2× SDS gel-loading buffer: 100 mM Tris–HCl pH 6.8, 4% (w/v) sodium dodecyl sulfate (or SDS, electrophoresis grade), 0.2% bromophenol blue, 20% (v/v) glycerol, 200 mM dithiothreitol (DTT) (*see* **Note 6**).

7. 10× SDS PAGE running buffer: Dissolve 30.0 g of Tris base, 144.0 g of glycine, and 10.0 g of SDS in 1 l of H_2O. This solution should have a pH of 8.3, but is expected that no pH adjustment will be required. Store the running buffer at room temperature and dilute to 1× before use (*see* **Note 7**).

8. Ethanol 70% (for cleaning the glass plates).

9. 10% SDS: dissolve 10 g of SDS in 80 ml H_2O. Complete volume to 100 ml. This solution can be kept at room temperature for up to 6 months.

2.3 Transfer

1. Nitrocellulose blotting membranes. We use 0.45 μm pore size for immunoblotting pRb, but a smaller pore size may be recommended should you want to adapt this protocol for low molecular weight proteins.

2. 1× transfer buffer: Dissolve 3.03 g Tris base and 14.4 g glycine in 500 ml H_2O. Add 200 ml methanol, and complete to a final volume of 1 l with dH_2O.

3. Tris-buffered saline with Tween 20 (TBST): First prepare a 10× TBS stock by dissolving 24.2 g of Tris base and 87.6 g NaCl in 800 ml H_2O, adjust to pH 7.6 with 1 M HCL, and complete to final volume of 1 l. To prepare the TBST, add 1 ml of Tween-20 to 1 l of 1× TBS.

4. Ponceau-S membrane staining solution: 0.5% (w/v) Ponceau-S in 1% acetic acid.

2.4 Immunoblotting Solutions and Antibodies

The protocols described in this chapter were optimized specifically for the antibodies described below and for several lung cancer cell lines.

1. Blocking solution: Dissolve 0.5 g of bovine serum albumin (BSA) in 10 ml of 1× TBST.

2. Primary antibody against phosphorylated serine 612 in pRb (anti-Rb Phospho-Ser612). We purchased this rabbit polyclonal antibody from Gene Tex (Cat. No. GTX24777), and use it at a dilution of 1:1000 in TBST. We usually prepare primary antibody solutions in TBTS that can be stored for several months at 4 °C. To prepare such antibody solutions, we dissolve 0.5 g of BSA in 10 ml of TBST, and add 30 μl of a 20% sodium azide stock. Sodium azide is used as a preservative to prevent bacterial growth in the solution. Sodium azide is toxic and a potential carcinogen, therefore, read carefully its accompanying Material Safety Data Sheet for information regarding proper handling, storage and disposal. Add 10 μl of the antibody to this solution. Mix and store at 4 °C. You can use this solution for several months, but you need to be attentive for signs of contamination such as a strong odor or cloudiness in the solution. In such case, discard and prepare a fresh solution. Use of contaminated antibody solution usually yields high background, meaning that it is time to replace the solution with a fresh one.

3. Primary antibody against phosphorylated threonine 821 (T821) in pRb (also rabbit monoclonal, Abcam Cat. No. ab32015). We prepare an antibody solution exactly as described above for the antibody against phospho-S612, except that for this antibody we use a dilution of 1:500. For this, we add 20 μl of antibody to the 10 ml TBST antibody solution including sodium azide as well.

4. Primary antibody against total pRb (mouse monoclonal 4H1, Cell Signaling Cat. No. 9309). We use at a dilution of 1:1000 in TBST, and we prepare it exactly as described above for the antibody against phospho-S612. It is important to blot for total pRb, as the extent of pRb phosphorylation is assessed and reported as the ratio of phosphorylated pRb to total pRb protein.

5. Secondary antibodies: we use horseradish peroxidase (HRP)-conjugated secondary antibodies. For mouse monoclonal primary antibodies, we use an HRP-conjugated, affinity-purified horse anti-mouse IgG (Cell Signaling, Cat. No. 7076S). For rabbit polyclonal primary antibodies, we use we use an HRP-conjugated, affinity-purified goat anti-rabbit IgG (Cell Signaling, Cat. No. 7074S). For both of these secondary antibodies, we prepare a TBST solution of the antibody exactly as described above for primary antibodies (except that we omit the sodium azide since we prepare fresh for each use), with the antibody diluted 1:5000.

6. Supersignal West Pico Plus™ Chemiluminescent Kit (Thermo Scientific Cat. No. 34078). This kit is compatible with HRP-conjugated secondary antibodies. The selection of the kit to develop the chemiluminescent signal is dictated by the enzyme conjugated to the secondary antibody (HRP, versus alkaline phosphatase, for example).

7. ChemiDoc imaging system and software, or other equivalent imaging system compatible with chemiluminescent signals.

2.5 Additional Equipment and Plasticware

1. Tabletop centrifuge with capacity for 15 ml tubes, preferably refrigerated.

2. 15 and 50 ml conical tubes.

3. Culture plates or bottles (we culture cells in T75 culture bottles).

4. Gel Electrophoresis system: parts and assembly as per manufacturer's instructions.

5. Transfer system: parts and assembly as per manufacturer's instructions.

6. 1.5 ml microcentrifuge tubes.

7. Refrigerated centrifuge for microcentrifuge tubes.

3 Methods

This protocol focuses on the immunoblot technique, and therefore it assumes that the user has cell cultures ready for protein extraction. We optimized the procedure described below using a variety of lung cancer cell lines, but this protocol is applicable to any pRb-expressing cell line in which pRb's phosphorylation status needs to be studied. It is important that you grow your cell cultures in the appropriate medium such that they are at approximately 90% confluence at the moment of protein extraction. This will ensure a good protein yield per plate, especially if you use large culture vessels such as T75 culture bottles.

3.1 Cell Lysis and Preparation of Protein Extracts

1. Collect cells by scrapping them from the culture plate in 2–3 ml of 1× PBS. We culture cells in T75 culture bottles, you should adjust the volume of PBS depending on your culture plate, but it is important to use the minimum volume of PBS that covers the entire culture surface. Alternatively, detach cells from the plate by incubating in trypsin–EDTA solution at 37 °C for 5 min (*see* **Note 8**).

2. Transfer the cell suspension to a 15 ml conical tube and pellet cells by low speed centrifugation (5 min at $400 \times g$). If you detach the cells using the trypsin EDTA solution, you need to dilute it 1:10 with culture medium to ensure inactivation of trypsin (before the centrifugation step). Remove the supernatant after the centrifugation.

3. Lyse cells by resuspending the cell pellet in RIPA buffer supplemented with proteases and phosphatase inhibitor cocktails (*see* **Note 9**). Transfer the cell suspension to a 1.5 ml microcentrifuge tube.

4. Incubate at 4 °C for 30 min to allow lysis to proceed (*see* **Note 10**).

5. Centrifuge tube for 10 min at $1400 \times g$ at 4 °C. Transfer supernatant to a fresh microcentrifuge tube.

6. Quantify the protein in your cell lysate using your method of choice (*see* **Note 11**).

3.2 SDS Polyacrylamide Gel Electrophoresis

1. Assemble your gel electrophoresis apparatus following manufacturer's instructions (*see* **Note 12**). At this point you will only need to assemble the gel casting system needed to pour the gels. We use a standard Bio-Rad gel electrophoresis apparatus with its accompanying gel casting system. Be sure to clean thoroughly all glass plates with 70% ethanol. This will ensure a smooth fingerprint-free glass surface, which will translate into decreased risk of forming bubbles while pouring the gel in between the glass plates.

2. Prepare the separating gel as follows: In a 50 ml conical tube, mix 7.9 ml of distilled water, 7 ml of the 30% acrylamide–bisacrylamide mix, 5.0 ml of 1.5 M Tris–HCl pH 8.8, 0.2 ml of 10% SDS. Add then 200 μl of 10% APS and 8 μl of TEMED. Gently mix avoiding as much as possible the formation of

bubbles. Keep in mind that the gel will start rapidly polymerizing after the addition of APS and TEMED, therefore these two reagents should be the very last to be added to the mix, and the gel should be poured immediately after their addition. Maintaining the mix on ice will also retard the polymerization (*see* **Notes 13** and **14**).

3. Allow the gel to completely polymerize for 30–60 min at room temperature (*see* **Note 15**). Be sure to always use freshly prepared or thawed APS (avoid refreezing of leftovers). Loss of APS activity is manifested in abnormally long polymerization times.

4. Prepare the upper stacking gel as follows: in a 15 ml conical tube, mix 4.1 ml of distilled H_2O, 1.0 ml of 30% acrylamide–bis-acrylamide mix, 750 μl of 0.5 M Tris–HCl pH 6.8, and 60 μl of 10% SDS. Mix gently avoiding foam and bubbles. When ready to pour, add 60 μl of 10% APS and 6 μl of TEMED. Mix and add it to the glass plates (*see* **Note 16**).

5. Immediately after pouring the stacking gel, insert comb being careful not to form any bubbles at the base of the wells. Allow the stacking gel to polymerize for 30–60 min at room temperature.

6. Carefully remove the comb and the bottom spacer. Please note that we do not recommend that you remove the comb straight out of the dry gel. Rather, we recommend that first you assemble the whole electrophoresis apparatus, including inserting the gel inside it, fill the liquid reservoir with running buffer, and then remove the comb. We use a standard protein gel electrophoresis apparatus from Bio-Rad. Dilute the 10× SDS PAGE running buffer to 1× with water and fill the assembled apparatus with it until you cover the gel. Only then we recommend that you slowly and carefully remove the comb (*see* **Note 17**). Using a glass or plastic Pasteur pipette, rinse the wells with running buffer to remove excess acrylamide.

7. Prepare the protein samples for loading into the gel. Mix enough volume of protein extract to contain 30–50 μg of total protein with an equal volume of 2× gel-loading buffer. Denature proteins by boiling the mixture at 95–100 °C for 5 min, or heating at 70 °C for 30 min.

8. Load the proteins into the wells, being careful not to over flood the wells (if you allow this to happen, you risk having a protein sample over flooding into an adjacent lane). Remember also to load a suitable protein ladder (*see* **Note 18**).

9. Place the lid on the electrophoresis apparatus, connect to a power supply, and run the gel at 160 V for 60 min (do not set a limit for Amperes). Monitor the run by following the bromophenol blue dye front. Stop the run when the dye front reaches about two-thirds of the length of the frontal glass plate (*see* **Note 19**).

3.3 Transfer of Proteins to Nitrocellulose Membranes

1. Disassemble the electrophoresis apparatus and remove the gel assembly. Very gently and carefully separate the glass plates from the gel carefully inserting a fine spatula in between the glass plates, and slowly twisting the spatula until the plates start to separate from the gel. Use a razor blade to carefully remove the stacking gel without damaging the separating gel. Rinse the gel with transfer buffer (*see* **Note 20**).

2. Cut a piece of nitrocellulose membrane of the approximate size of the gel (a little bit larger so you can handle it by the edges without touching the gel) and immerse in cold transfer buffer for 2–5 min (*see* **Note 21**).

3. Prewet several pieces of filter paper (cut in a size similar to the gel) in cold transfer buffer by submerging one side of the paper first and then slowly lowering it into the buffer.

4. Assemble the gel electrotransfer cassette following the manufacturer's instructions (*see* **Notes 22** and **23**).

5. Insert the transfer cassette into the electrotransfer unit. It is usual for electro-transfer units to have a special compartment for an ice block or any other cooling device. As the transfer process generates heat and the transfer buffer can get warm (or even hot), it is recommended that the ice block/cooling devices are used (*see* **Note 24**).

6. Transfer for 60 min at 100 V (do not set a limit for Amperes).

7. After the transfer is completed, disassemble the unit. Wash the membrane in TBST to remove residual SDS and potential gel fragments.

8. Check the efficiency of transfer by staining the membrane in Ponceau-S solution for 5 min at room temperature. Ponceau-stained membranes can be seen in Fig. 1a, b (*see* **Note 25**). Record an image of the Ponceau-stained membrane using a document scanner or camera. Never let membranes to get dry. Keep membranes moist during the documentation process by keeping them wrapped in plastic wrap after soaking in transfer buffer. *See* **Notes 26–28** for transfer troubleshooting tips.

3.4 Immunoblotting, Image Development and Capture

1. Remove the Ponceau-S staining from the membrane by incubating in TBST containing 5% milk. You will notice the milk solution turning red. Discard and rinse the membrane with TBST (no milk). Repeat until no trace of the red Ponceau-S stain remains in the membrane. At this point you should only see the rainbow-colored protein markers. Repeat a final rinse with TBST (*see* **Note 29**).

2. Block membranes in TBST with BSA (*see* **Note 29**). You can block for 2 h at room temperature or overnight at 4 °C. Use constant agitation to ensure that the membrane is constantly bathed by the solution.

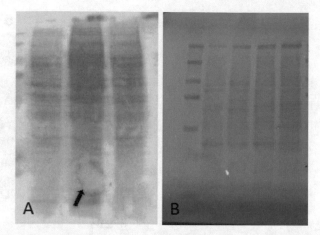

Fig. 1 Representative membranes stained with Ponceau-S stain. (**a**) This membrane shows unequal loading of the lanes, as it can be appreciated that the middle lane has a higher amount of protein compared to the lanes at the sides. A clear protein-less spot can be seen in the bottom part of the middle lane (arrow). This effect was likely generated by a bubble being trapped between the gel and the membrane during the transfer process. (**b**) This membrane shows similar protein loading in the lanes, no air bubble marks, and no signs of protein degradation, which are usually seen as a low molecular weight diffuse smear in the lower half of the membrane

3. Incubate membranes with the primary antibody. Like the blocking step, primary antibody incubation can be done either 2 h at room temperature, or overnight at 4 °C. Use constant agitation during this step as well (*see* **Note 30**).

4. Wash three times in TBST.

5. Incubate with secondary antibody for 1 h at room temperature while agitating (*see* **Note 31**).

6. For development of the membrane chemiluminescence, we use the Supersignal West Pico Plus™ Chemiluminescent Kit (Thermo Scientific Cat. No. 34580), following the procedures exactly as described by the manufacturer. We add 1 ml of substrate solution per membrane. Do not leave it for more than 3 min (*see* **Note 32**).

7. Capture the chemiluminescent signal using a ChemiDoc imaging system or its equivalent (we use ChemiDoc XRS+), using the accompanying image software for image capturing and quantification of signal intensity. A typical immunoblot result using this protocol is shown in Fig. 2a. Notice that you need to run in parallel immunoblots using the phospho-specific antibodies as well as antibodies recognizing total pRb protein. You need to assess pRb phosphorylation in the residues of your interest relative to total pRb levels, in other words, as the ratio of phosphorylated pRb to total pRb (Fig. 2a, b) (*see* **Note 33**).

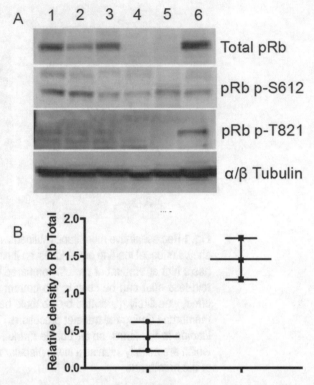

Fig. 2 Typical immunoblot analysis of different lung cancer cell lines (lanes 1–6) using antibodies against phosphorylated pRb residues S162 and T821, as well as against total pRb. (**a**) Except for cell lines in lanes 4 and 5, all other cell lines express endogenous pRb. Notice that cell lines in lanes 1–3 and 6 express total pRb as well as showing pRb phosphorylation in serine 612. On the other hand, of these 4 cell lines, the one in lane 6 is the only one showing hyperphosphorylation in threonine 821. (**b**) After densitometric analysis of band intensity for signal quantification, we determined the ratio of signal intensity of pRb phospho-T821 to total pRb levels. The graph shows the phosphorylation in T821 as a fraction of total pRb for cell lines in lanes 1 and 6. Serine 821 is hyperphosphorylated in 6 relative to 1 in a statistically significant manner (p value = 0.007)

---

4 Notes

1. Given that pRb is an intranuclear antigen, detaching the cells with trypsin is acceptable. There are many suppliers for trypsin-EDTA solutions which are sold as a 10× stock that require a 1:10 dilution before using. Ready-to-use trypsin-EDTA solutions are also available. The important aspect to consider is that you should aim for a final concentration of 0.05% trypsin and 0.02% EDTA. Also, if adding the trypsin solution, you need to wash the culture plate with PBS before the trypsin step to ensure that you completely remove the culture medium which may contain trypsin inhibitors.

2. Protease inhibitors in the cell lysis buffer minimize protein degradation during extraction. We use Protease Inhibitor Cocktail from Sigma-Aldrich (Cat. No. P8340-5ML). Phosphatase inhibitors are particularly important in this protocol; keep in mind that you want to assess pRb's phosphorylation status, therefore inhibition of the endogenous phosphatases is of paramount importance. If you use the $10\times$ RIPA buffer from Cell Signaling (Cat. No. 9806), it already includes the phosphatase inhibitors 2.5 mM sodium pyrophosphate and 1 mM sodium orthovanadate (Na_3VO_4). If you do not use the Cell Signaling premixed RIPA buffer, you can purchase these phosphatase inhibitors separately and add them to the RIPA buffer at the moment of use, making sure you use them at the final concentrations indicated above.

3. When adjusting pH with HCL, you can start with concentrated HCL (e.g., 12 M), but then change to a more diluted acid (e.g., 1 M) as you get closer to the desired pH.

4. You can also prepare this solution by diluting the 1.5 M Tris–HCl stock and adjusting the pH.

5. We use the premixed Bio-Rad (Cat. No. 161-0158, keep stored at 4 °C), but you can try other options.

6. You can prepare this solution from the Tris–HCl pH 6.8 stock and a 10% SDS stock. 200 mM beta-mercaptoethanol (BME) can be used in place of DTT as a reducing agent to break disulfide bonds. Without the reducing agent (DTT or BME), this buffer can be stored at room temperature. Add the DTT from a 1 M stock, and use the solution right after adding the DTT. If pipetting concentrated glycerol becomes difficult, you can cut the pipette tip.

7. For convenience, Bio-Rad has a premade $1\times$ SDS PAGE running buffer (Cat. No. 161-0732), but preparing this buffer from common laboratory reagents should work well.

8. Avoid overtrypsinization as it may kill cells. Fresh trypsin solution should detach cells in under 5 min. If you find that 5 min under trypsin-EDTA are not enough to detach cells from the plate, it is better to get a fresh trypsin-EDTA batch than prolonging the trypsinization time.

9. It is recommended that you obtain an estimate of the number of cells per plate (using any common procedure such as trypan blue exclusion staining) before extracting proteins from each plate. This information is useful since we recommend that you lyse cells in 200 μl of RIPA buffer per 10^6 cells. To minimize protein degradation, lysis should be conducted using cold solutions, and keeping cells on ice as much as possible during the process.

10. During those 30 min, you can enhance the amount of proteins released by cells by passing the lysate 3–5 times through a syringe with a 27.5-gauge needle. While this significantly increases protein yield, it could also produce foaming, which should be avoided to prevent protein loss.

11. We perform a standard protein quantification assay using Bio-Rad's Protein Assay (Cat. No. 500-0006), following its instructions, and using BSA as a quantification standard. Other substitute assays can be used. After quantification, protein lysates that will not be used immediately can be stored at −20 °C for up to 3 months (protein integrity cannot be ensured beyond that).

12. Choose the number of wells according to your number of samples and experimental design. Regarding the thickness of the gel (this is determined by the thickness of the spacers that you use), a thicker gel will allow you to load a larger sample volume, which is a necessity if your protein sample is not very concentrated. This, however, can adversely affect the efficiency of the transfer, high molecular weight proteins being particularly affected. For that reason, aim to get as concentrated as possible protein samples, in order to be able to load smaller volumes on the gel. Be aware then, that thinner gels require extra caution when handling, as they are prone to break apart during handling.

13. It is recommended that you add a thin layer of isopropanol on top of the separating gel solution immediately after pouring it. Isopropanol is not miscible in water, thus it will form a distinct layer. Adding isopropanol eliminates any bubbles on the surface of the separating gel solution and will produce a smooth surface. As an alternative, we use the premixed gel system 10% SDS-PAGE FastCast acrylamide starter kit (Cat. No. 1610172) from Bio-Rad. This kit contains the buffers for the separating and stacking gels, and has a considerably reduced time for polymerization.

14. For pRb, which has a molecular weight of approximately 110 kDa, we use a 10% polyacrylamide separating gel. The % of polyacrylamide you will choose depends on the molecular weight range in which you want to have good resolution. Take this into consideration if you wish to adapt this protocol to other phosphoproteins.

15. After 45 min, you can verify if the gel has polymerized by *gently* tilting the casting apparatus sideways. Only the isopropanol layer should move while the underlying separating gel should be static if it has polymerized.

16. To save time, you can start preparing the stacking gel while the separating gel is polymerizing. However, *do not add the*

TEMED and the APS until immediately before adding the stacking gel to the casting apparatus. The stacking gel without APS and TEMED can be kept on ice until pouring. The % of acrylamide of the stacking gel is usually smaller (4–6%) than that of the separating gel.

17. If you slowly remove the comb having the gel submerged in running buffer, you will notice that as you remove the comb the empty well space is immediately filled with buffer. This will avoid the collapse of the well that is experienced if you remove the comb out of the dry gel, as a vacuum is formed inside the well as the comb is retrieved.

18. When blotting for pRb, we use Bio-Rad Precision Plus Protein Kaleidoscope (Cat. No. 1610-375). You can use any other protein ladder provided it has sufficient markers in the molecular weight range of your protein of interest, in this case, around 110 kDa, which is the approximate molecular weight of pRb.

19. Running time depends on gel thickness. Here we used 1.5 mm gels. If you notice a distortion of band shapes ("smiley bands"), decrease the voltage. Be careful to stop the run when the tracking dye has reached two-thirds of the way, otherwise you risk losing low molecular weight proteins. This may not be an issue with pRb, but is an issue to consider if you want to adapt this protocol to study other proteins.

20. This is a very sensitive step; if not done carefully, you risk breaking the gel apart. Remember that the thinner the gel, the higher the risk of this occurring. Never let the gel get dry. Keep it soaked from here on in transfer buffer.

21. Always handle the membrane with gloves or with tweezers. Never touch the membrane with bare hands, this may leave fingerprints oils on the membrane and this in turn will prevent even wetting of the membrane. This usually results in areas in the membrane where transfer of proteins is impaired.

22. It is difficult on this step to elaborate on the specifics of the assembly of the electro-transfer transfer cassette and unit as this depends on the specific model and vendor. However, regardless of the apparatus that you use, it is very important that you are mindful of the direction in which the proteins will flow. Due to the SDS in the sample buffer, proteins will be negatively charged, and therefore they will move toward the positive pole in an electrical field. Therefore, the membrane must be positioned between the gel and the positive pole. This will make the proteins become attached to the membrane as they transit to the positive pole.

23. When assembling the transfer unit, it is extremely important that you avoid at all costs the formation of bubbles between

the gel and the membrane. A place where a bubble is formed is a place where transfer of proteins will be affected.

24. The transfer can be done in a cold room, or the whole transfer apparatus can be inserted in a tray and surrounded with ice during the transfer process.

25. We strongly recommend that you stain the membrane after transfer with Ponceau-S stain. This procedure is highly informative, as it will allow you to assess whether you loaded approximately equal amounts of total protein in all wells, and if you obtained an even and efficient transfer of proteins (Fig. 1a–b). Usually places where bubbles formed (or transfer did not occur due to any other reason) can be seen in the stained membrane as protein-free clear areas. The decision of whether it is worth proceeding to subsequent steps can usually be done after assessing the quality of transfer in a Ponceau-S stained membrane. Poor transfer is usually the culprit of most problems commonly encountered in this technique.

26. Do not exceed the transfer time as this leads to gel shrinkage and distortion of the membrane. In case of poor transfer efficiency, opt for making thinner gels, rather that prolonging transfer time.

27. If there are unstained "white spots" on the membrane seen after Ponceau-S staining, this may have been caused by air bubbles trapped between the gel and the membrane. Make sure to remove all the bubbles when preparing the transfer cassette. An air bubble does not necessarily ruin an experiment; it depends on its size and on the molecular weight range in which it formed. If your protein of interest is not in this range, you may choose to proceed with the subsequent steps.

28. Ponceau-S staining may also help you to spot degraded proteins, which are appreciated as a diffuse smear in the lower half on the membrane. In this case, ensure that you are taking all the precautions necessary to deal with protein degradation, such as not using protein samples that have been stored for prolonged times (or repeatedly frozen-thawed), ensuring that cell lysis was done on ice and the samples were kept cold or refrigerated all the times, and that you added protease inhibitors to the RIPA buffer.

29. When doing a western blot using antibodies against phosphorylated residues, it is important that you thoroughly remove any traces on milk from the membrane. Casein (milk protein) is heavily phosphorylated and any traces of milk in the membrane can lead to high background due to nonspecific antibody binding. For the same reason, the blocking solution must not contain milk. The blocking step is usually one of the steps in which you can make adjustments in case you experience high background levels.

30. Incubating in primary antibody for 2 h versus overnight must be empirically determined. Longer incubation periods are recommended if you are having trouble obtaining strong signals. However, be aware that longer incubation times also increase the likelihood of obtaining a strong background. The length of the incubation time (with primary antibody) is one of the factors that affect signal strength. Dilution of antibody also usually affects background noise. If you are obtaining too much background, in addition to extending blocking time, you can try diluting the primary antibody. Conversely, try concentrating the primary antibody if you obtain weak signals.

31. Ensure that the secondary antibody is properly chosen to match the primary antibody. For example, if you use a mouse primary antibody, the secondary antibody must be a goat anti-mouse or donkey anti-mouse antibody. Incompatibility between primary and secondary antibody is a usual source or mistakes in this technique.

32. Other commercially available kits can be acceptable substitutes, as long as they are compatible with the enzyme that is conjugated to the secondary antibody. The signal development step also has a major impact on signal intensity and background. This step can be performed for 30 s to 3 min. If you are experiencing weak signals, in addition to using more concentrated primary antibody and/or increasing incubation time, you can try developing the membrane for longer (but do not exceed 3 min, as this may blacken the membrane). Some antibodies give a very strong signal and in such cases, 30 s to 1 min is sufficient.

33. As part of the optimization of phospho-specific antibodies, it is important that you ensure that they are indeed detecting the phosphorylated residues of interest. A simple way to verify this is to conduct initial experiments in which you treat protein extracts with calf intestinal phosphatase (treat with 50 units of phosphatase per 50 μg of total protein, 37 °C overnight). This treatment should eliminate immunoreactivity if the antibody is indeed recognizing a phosphorylated form of the protein of interest. Remember to include controls treated with phosphatase buffer alone, as well as a control with phosphatase in the presence of phosphatase inhibitors.

References

1. Weinberg RA (1995) The Rb protein and cell cycle control. Cell 81:323–330
2. Dyson N (1998) The regulation of E2F by pRB-family proteins. Genes Dev 12: 2245–2262
3. Thomas DM, Carty SA, Piscopo DM, Lee J-S, Wang W-F et al (2001) The retinoblastoma protein acts as a transcriptional coactivator required for osteogenic differentiation. Mol Cell 8:303–316

4. Knudsen ES, Knudsen KE (2006) Retinoblastoma tumor suppressor: where cancer meets cell cycle. Exp Biol Med 231: 1271–1281

5. Rubin SM (2013) Deciphering the retinoblastoma protein phosphorylation code. Trends Biochem Sci 38(1):12–19

6. Lundberg AS, Weinberg RA (1998) Functional inactivation of the retinoblastoma protein requires sequential modification by at least two distinct cyclin-cdk complexes. Mol Cell Biol 18(2):753–761

7. Diehl JA (2002) Cycling to cancer with cyclin D1. Cancer Biol Ther 3:226–231

8. Burke JR, Liban TJ, Restrepo T, Lee HW, Rubin SM (2014) Multiple mechanisms for E2F binding inhibition by phosphorylation of the retinoblastoma protein C-terminal domain. J Mol Biol 426(1):245–255

9. Munro S, Carr SM, La Thangue NB (2012) Diversity within the pRb pathway: is there a code of conduct? Oncogene 31(40):4343

10. Hattori T, Uchida C, Takahashi H, Yamamoto N, Naito M, Taya Y (2014) Distinct and site-specific phosphorylation of the retinoblastoma protein at serine 612 in differentiated cells. PLoS One 9(1):e86709

11. Lentine B, Antonucci L, Hunce R, Edwards J, Marallano V, Krucher NA (2012) Dephosphorylation of threonine-821 of the retinoblastoma tumor suppressor protein (Rb) is required for apoptosis induced by UV and Cdk inhibition. Cell Cycle 11(17):3324–3330

12. MacDonald JI, Dick FA (2012) Posttranslational modifications of the retinoblastoma tumor suppressor protein as determinants of function. Genes Cancer 3(11-12): 619–633

Chapter 7

Immunohistochemical Detection of the Retinoblastoma Protein

Charles A. Ishak, Matthew J. Cecchini, Christopher J. Howlett, and Frederick A. Dick

Abstract

The retinoblastoma protein (pRB) plays a key role in proliferative control and genome stability. For these reasons its functions are considered to be tumor suppressive. Its functional status offers critical insight into proliferative control signaling in tissues and in developing malignancies. In this chapter, we outline basic procedures to detect the retinoblastoma protein in formalin fixed, paraffin embedded tissue sections. In addition, we provide protocols to detect phosphorylation levels of pRB in tissues and offer controls to ensure fidelity of measurement. Importantly, these staining methods utilize broadly available reagents and equipment making them accessible to most biomedical research laboratories.

Key words Cell cycle, Phosphorylation, Cancer, Immunohistochemistry, Retinoblastoma protein

1 Introduction

The retinoblastoma susceptibility gene (*RB1*) was first discovered for its role in a rare pediatric cancer. Since its initial discovery, the protein encoded by *RB1* (pRB) has been demonstrated to be widely expressed among human tissues [1]. The pRB protein is phosphorylated by Cyclin-Dependent Kinases (CDKs) at the onset of S-phase and it remains phosphorylated until late in mitosis when it is dephosphorylated [2]. The pRB protein exists in a state of low phosphorylation in G1 where it binds to E2F family transcription factors. At the onset of S-phase it is extensively phosphorylated and E2Fs are released to activate transcription and advance the cell cycle. Data suggest that most human cancers express a wild type pRB protein, but contain alterations that misregulate CDKs, leading to elevated pRB phosphorylation and deregulated cell cycle entry [3]. From this perspective, the detection of pRB and its relative phosphorylation level offers insights into proliferative control status because these measurements can be related directly to cell cycle control mechanisms.

Pedro G. Santiago-Cardona (ed.), *The Retinoblastoma Protein*, Methods in Molecular Biology, vol. 1726, https://doi.org/10.1007/978-1-4939-7565-5_7, © Springer Science+Business Media, LLC 2018

Immunohistochemical analysis of pRB and its phosphorylation status offers a number of means to obtain valuable information about the tissue or tumor in question. In particular, pRB positivity in immunohistochemical analysis has been shown to offer prognostic significance that may be used to predict responsiveness to different therapies [4–6]. In addition, new targeted agents have been developed to inhibit Cyclin D associated CDKs and the best prediction of response to these agents is the phosphorylation status of pRB [7]. Thus, immunohistochemical detection of pRB and its relative phosphorylation status offers a number of opportunities to enhance insight into tumor biology and drug responsiveness.

In this chapter, we outline a protocol for immunohistochemical detection of pRB. We use this approach for standard detection of pRB in a formalin-fixed, paraffin-embedded (FFPE) tissue section. We have used this to examine relative expression levels of pRB in human lung and ovarian tumors from archival tissue samples [4]. Based on the broad species specificity of the G3-245 monoclonal antibody against pRB chosen for these studies, we expect this methodology to be applicable to studies of pRB in tissues from mice and other mammals. We also include methodology for detecting relative phosphorylation of pRB at S807 and S811. This is an excellent companion to the detection of overall pRB levels as it helps to guide conclusions on the cell cycle arrest activity that pRB may be exerting in the tissue at the time of fixation.

As with most histological analyses, these methods work best with high quality specimens. Investigators should be cautious to ensure that tissues are fixed with sufficiently abundant volumes of formalin to ensure rapid and thorough fixation. Inadequate fixation will lead to tissue degradation and uninterpretable staining and cellular architecture. Similarly, excessively long fixation will prevent antigen retrieval and tissues will become brittle. Following chemical processing and embedding of tissues, the quality of sections cut from a microtome will have significant impact on the quality of data, as uneven thickness or tears in the section will lead to differential staining intensity. Lastly, image capture can greatly affect the quality of data. While a high-quality camera mounted on a standard upright microscope is sufficient to generate reliable images, new slide scanning automated microscopes can standardize much of these procedures and remove inconsistencies introduced by investigators.

2 Materials

All solutions should be made with ultrapure water with particular attention paid to potential sources of phosphatase activity that may be found in blocking agents or in older, microbiologically contaminated solutions. Care should be taken to properly dispose of toxic solvents according to institutional guidelines.

2.1 Solvents and Solutions

1. Citrate Buffer: 10 mM Na-citrate, pH 6.0. To prepare 1 L, dissolve 2.94 g of trisodium citrate dehydrate in 1 L H_2O, and adjust the pH to 6.0 with 1 N HCl.

2. Tris Buffered Saline (TBS): 20 mM Tris, pH 7.5, 150 mM NaCl. Prepare a 10× stock by dissolving 24 g of Tris base and 88 g of NaCl in 900 mL distilled H_2O. Bring to pH 7.5 with 12 N HCl, and complete to 1 L with distilled H_2O. For a 1× solution, dilute 1 part 10× stock with 9 parts of distilled H_2O, adjust pH again to 7.5.

3. Dulbecco's Phosphate Buffered Saline (PBS): 10 mM Phosphate, pH 7.4, 137 mM NaCl, 2.7 mM KCl. The standard recipe for 1 L of 1× PBS consists of 8 g NaCl, 0.2 g KCl, 1.44 g Na_2HPO_4, and 0.24 g KH_2PO_4. Dissolve in 800 mL H_2O, adjust pH to 7.4 with HCL, and complete final volume of 1 L with H_2O. Dispense into aliquots and sterilize either by autoclaving (20 min at 15 PSI) or by filtering.

4. Tris Buffered Saline–Tween (TBS-T): TBS with 0.2% Tween 20.

5. Phosphate Buffered Saline–Tween (PBS-T): PBS with 0.2% Tween 20.

6. Xylene: ACS reagent grade xylenes.

7. Ethanol: 100%, 95%, and 70% either purchased or diluted with ddH_2O.

8. Blocking Solution: 10% Goat Serum in TBS-T.

9. Peroxide Blocking Solution: 3% H_2O_2 in PBS.

10. Hematoxylin Solution: Mayer's hematoxylin 1 g/L in H_2O.

2.2 Antibodies and Other Commercial Reagents

1. Lambda protein phosphatase and buffer: We purchase Lambda phosphatase along with a 10× Protein MetalloPhosphatase (PMP) buffer stock (once diluted to 1×, this buffer consists of 50 mM HEPES, 100 mM NaCL, 2 mM DTT, 0.01% Brij 35, pH 7.5 at 25 °C), and a 10× stock of 10 mM $MnCl_2$ that is an essential cofactor.

2. Anti-pRB antibodies: We use mouse anti-pRB monoclonal G3-245 (Cat. No. 554136, BD Biosciences) diluted 1:300 in Blocking Solution. This antibody produces the most reliable results and is the standard for pRB detection.

3. Anti-pS807/pS811 pRB antibodies: We use a rabbit polyclonal antibody directed against this modification from Cell Signaling Technologies (Cat. No. 9308, Cell Signaling) diluted 1:200 in Blocking Solution. We have found this to be the most reliable source for this phosphospecific antibody.

4. Anti-mouse secondary antibody: Biotinylated Goat anti-mouse IgG secondary antibody diluted 1:200 in Blocking Solution.

5. Anti-rabbit secondary antibody: Biotinylated Goat anti-rabbit IgG secondary antibody diluted 1:200 in Blocking Solution.

6. Streptavidin-HRP: We prefer a ready to use stock already diluted in the appropriate buffer for binding the biotinylated secondary antibody.

7. DAB HRP substrate: We purchase DAB as a stock solution accompanied by the appropriate diluent buffer for use.

8. Mounting Medium: We use VectaMount Permanent Mounting Medium.

2.3 Equipment and Supplies

1. Microwavable pressure cooker or equivalent.

2. Stainless steel microscope slide rack and glass staining dish.

3. Plastic Coplin jars.

4. Forceps for handling glass slides.

5. Absorbent low lint tissues (e.g., Kimwipes).

6. Hydrophobic barrier pen for circling mounted tissue sections on glass slides.

7. Humidified chamber for slide staining. We typically use 15 cm plastic cell culture dishes containing a moist paper towel. A sealable plastic food storage container with a moist paper towel on the bottom will work similarly.

8. Orbital platform shaker with variable speed control.

3　Methods

Immunohistochemical techniques are relatively ubiquitous and the methods outlined below follow relatively standard methods. We commonly use an institutional service for tissue processing, embedding, sectioning, and have standard 4 μm thick tissue sections mounted on 26 × 76 mm charged glass slides. For this reason, we do not provide methods for these steps. We refer investigators to other sources for these protocols [8]. Detection of pRB by immunohistochemistry is shown in Fig. 1 and demonstrates the range of staining intensities that are typical using this approach.

We have also used antibodies directed against pRB that recognize phosphorylation on S807 and S811. Antibodies that detect these sites were selected because in our experience these are the most reliable phosphospecific antibodies against pRB [9–11]. In general, pRB is inactive for cell cycle control functions when extensively phosphorylated, however, we caution users of our methods that phosphorylation of these two sites alone cannot fully explain pRB's functional status [2]. We selected antibodies based

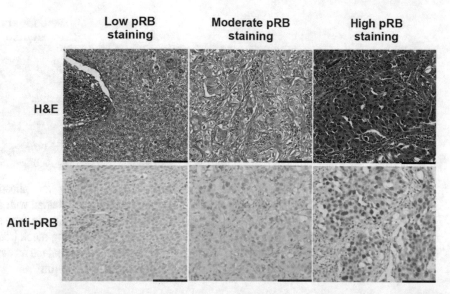

Fig. 1 Lung adenocarcinomas stained for pRB. Sections were stained with Hematoxylin and Eosin to reveal tissue architecture (top). Consecutive sections of the same specimen were also stained for pRB by immuno-histochemistry (bottom). Shown is an example of low pRB staining that is consistent with a genetic deficiency for the RB1 gene (leftmost sample). A moderately stained sample shows staining intensity for pRB that is similar between stromal cells and tumor cells in the same tissue section (center). Lastly, unusually high staining for pRB is shown (right). Note that staining intensity of tumor cells exceed that of the surrounding stroma. Scale bars represent 100 μm

on specificity that is borne out in western blotting experiments (phosphospecific antibodies against S807 and S811 generally have few cross reacting bands), we have also used lambda phosphatase treatment to quality control specimen staining to ensure that the signal is dependent on phosphorylation (Fig. 2). We suggest that this type of analysis of pRB phosphorylation could be expanded to other phosphorylation sites provided control experiments for antibody specificity are included.

3.1 Deparaffinization and Rehydration of Slide-Mounted Sections

1. In a fume hood, prepare three glass staining dishes containing 500 mL of xylene (*see* **Note 1**).

2. Similarly, prepare two glass staining dishes containing 500 mL of each of the following: 100% ethanol, 95% ethanol, 70% ethanol, and ddH$_2$O.

3. Place slides in a stainless-steel rack such that tissue sections on each slide all project in the same orientation.

4. Submerge rack and slides into the first 500 mL xylene bath and incubate for 5 min.

5. Repeat the 5 min incubation in **step 4** in the second and then third xylene baths. The sections are now deparaffinized.

6. Transfer rack with deparaffinized sections into the first 100% ethanol bath and incubate for 3 min.

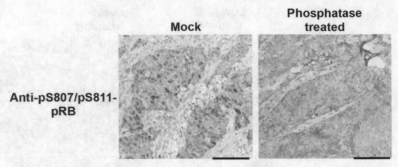

Fig. 2 High grade serous ovarian tumors stained for phosphorylated pRB. Consecutive sections from the same sample were stained with antibodies directed to pRB phosphorylated on S807 and S811. The samples were stained as described in this protocol with the sample on the left being mock treated while the sample on the right was digested with lambda phosphatase as described in Subheading 3.5 of this protocol. Scale bars represent 100 μm

7. Transfer the rack to the second 100% ethanol bath and incubate for 3 min.

8. Repeat **steps 6** and **7**, first in the 90% ethanol baths, followed by the 70% ethanol baths.

9. Transfer the rack into the first ddH$_2$O bath and place under a running tap of dH$_2$O for 3 min in a sink. Take care to ensure that water is not pouring directly onto tissue sections but is instead entering at the edge of the dish to circulate dH$_2$O around the tissue sections.

10. Transfer the rack into the second ddH$_2$O bath and repeat **step 9**.

3.2 Blocking Endogenous Peroxidase Activity of Rehydrated Tissue

1. Fill a plastic slide chamber with 100 mL Peroxide Blocking Solution (*see* **Note 1**).

2. Using forceps, transfer slides from the stainless-steel rack into the slide chamber taking care to only handle the slides by the edges so that the tissue section is unperturbed. Place all slides in the chamber in the same orientation so that tissue sections are not able to contact one another.

3. Incubate sections for 10 min.

4. Carefully discard Peroxide Blocking Solution and replace with 100 mL of PBS. Take care to ensure that PBS is not poured directly on tissue sections as this can compromise tissue architecture.

5. Repeat **step 4** with another PBS wash and incubate for 1 min.

3.3   Heat-Induced Antigen Retrieval

1. Fill a plastic Coplin jar with 100 mL of Citrate Buffer (*see* **Note 1**).

2. Use forceps to transfer slides into jar with Citrate Buffer.

3. Place jar in center of pressure cooker and add Citrate Buffer until it is ¼ submerged.

4. Seal pressure cooker and microwave at full power for 15 min, this will ensure that the buffer boils for a prolonged period of time (*see* **Note 2**)

5. Upon completion, carefully remove pressure cooker, wait until cooled (approximately 30 min), then release pressure. Remove Coplin jar from pressure cooker and leave on bench top until it has cooled to room temperature.

3.4   Blocking of Nonspecific Antibody Binding

1. Replace Citrate Buffer with 100 mL of PBS-T. Gently agitate for 1 min on an orbital shaker at 15 revolutions per minute (rpm).

2. Replace with fresh PBS-T, and repeat **step 1**.

3. Remove slides from the jar one at a time. Drain buffer from the slide by holding one end and carefully remove buffer around tissue using a Kimwipes. Do not touch the tissue section with the Kimwipes.

4. Encircle tissue with a hydrophobic pen and allow hydrophobic barrier to dry for 30 s.

5. Place slide in a humidified container and pipette 200 μL of Blocking Solution to cover tissue within hydrophobic barrier (*see* **Note 3**). Close cover to humidified chamber and incubate for 1 h.

6. Repeat **steps 3–5** for each slide.

3.5   Phosphatase-Based Validation of Phosphospecific Staining

1. Once slides have been blocked for nonspecific antibody binding, they can be returned to a plastic Coplin jar and washed in PBS-T for 5 min (*see* **Note 4**).

2. Lay slides flat in humidified chamber and Pipette 200 μL of 1× PMP buffer containing 1 mM $MnCl_2$ and 4000 units of Lambda phosphatase onto each desired slide.

3. Pipette 200 μL of 1× PMP buffer containing 1 mM $MnCl_2$ onto control slides in a humidified chamber to be used as a mock phosphatase control.

4. Close the humidified chamber and incubate at 37 °C for 1 h.

3.6   Immunostaining of Exposed Antigens with Primary Antibody (Anti-pRB, or Anti-pS807/S811 pRB)

1. Prepare sufficient volume of primary antibody dilutions in Blocking Solution to ensure 200 μL is available for each slide.

2. Designate one slide to omit from primary antibody immunostaining as an antibody specificity control.

3. For all other slides, gently drain blocking buffer from slide by tipping on end.

4. Carefully pipette 200 μL of primary antibody dilution onto tissue within enclosed hydrophobic barrier.

5. Close humidified container and incubate primary antibody overnight at 4 °C. For the unstained control, continue to incubate the slide overnight in Blocking Solution and process it alongside all others in the subsequent sections of this protocol.

3.7 Immunostaining with Secondary Antibody

1. Carefully remove primary antibody dilution from each slide.

2. Transfer slides from humidified container into plastic slide chamber containing 100 mL of PBS-T and gently agitate on rotating platform at 15 rpm for 5 min.

3. Replace PBS-T and repeat gentle shaking for 5 min. Repeat this step for a total of three PBS-T washes.

4. Prepare a 1:200 dilution of secondary antibody conjugated to biotin in Blocking Solution. Use anti-mouse secondary for detecting the murine derived G3-245 primary antibody against pRB and the anti-rabbit secondary for detecting the phosphospecific anti-pS807/pS811 pRB antibody that was generated in rabbits. Pipette 200 μL of secondary antibody dilution onto tissue within enclosed hydrophobic barrier. Incubate for 1 h in a closed humidified container at room temperature.

5. Carefully remove secondary antibody dilution from slides.

6. Transfer slides from humidified container into plastic Coplin jar containing 100 mL of PBS-T and gently agitate on rotating platform at 15 rpm for 5 min. Repeat two more times for three washes total.

7. Remove slides from chamber, apply 1 drop of ready to use streptavidin-HRP (approximately 200 μL) to cover tissue and incubate in a closed humidified container for 30 min at room temperature.

8. Remove streptavidin-HRP solution and place slides into Coplin jar containing 100 mL of TBS. Rotate on platform for 5 min as before and repeat TBS washes two more times for three washes total.

9. Prepare DAB solution by diluting 1 drop into 1 mL of diluent (as per manufacturer's instructions).

10. Remove slides from jar, lay them down flat, and gently cover tissue with 200 μL DAB solution. Incubate for 5 min at room temperature to permit chromogenic development (*see* **Note 5**).

11. Remove DAB solution. Wash slides twice in Coplin jar with 100 mL of PBS-T each time. Agitate on rotating platform for 2 min during each wash.

12. Carefully drain PBS-T and replace with ddH$_2$O. Rotate on platform for an additional 2 min.

3.8 Staining with Hematoxylin and Dehydration of Tissue

1. Remove slides from chamber and place on flat surface. Pipette 200 μL of Hematoxylin Solution onto tissue and incubate for 5 min at room temperature.

2. Transfer slides into a stainless-steel slide holder as before and submerge in a glass staining dish containing tap water. Place in a sink and rinse under a gentle but steady source of running water for 5 min.

3. Transfer slides in stainless steel rack to a 95% ethanol bath and incubate for 2 min.

4. Transfer slides to a second 95% ethanol bath, and repeat 2 min incubation.

5. Transfer slides to a 100% ethanol bath and incubate for 3 min.

6. Move slides to a second 100% ethanol bath and incubate for 3 min.

7. Remove slide rack and allow excess ethanol to drain.

8. Lay slides flat on bench top and apply three drops of Mounting Medium to tissue and apply coverslip at an angle, slowly lower the coverslip to avoid trapping air bubbles.

9. Incubate for 1 h at room temperature until mounting medium is dried.

4 Notes

1. We use large glass dishes with approximately 20 slide capacity stainless steel racks to transfer slides between dishes. In cases where tissue microarrays are being stained, smaller dishes that hold fewer slides may be preferable and the volumes of solvent can be scaled down as required. Similarly, our solution volumes for Coplin jars are based on the items we use, but these can be readily adjusted to suit any scale of staining, or type of container. Regardless of containers and buffer volumes, it is critical that slides are fully submerged for all steps described that use glass staining dishes or plastic Coplin jars.

2. Due to variable performance of different microwaves the time indicated is a good starting point for most experiments, but this step may need to be optimized by different investigators.

3. The amount of solution needed to completely cover the tissue specimen mounted on the slide is very much dependent on the size of the section and the area demarcated by the hydrophobic pen. For us 200 μL is typically sufficient, but investigators should ensure that sufficient quantity of buffer is used such that the sample is completely covered with buffer. The Blocking Solution and procedures described are optimized for staining human tissue. Blocking protocols may need to be varied for other species, particularly mouse tissues where anti-mouse secondary antibodies can readily detect endogenous immunoglobulins.

4. The methods described in Subheading 3.5 are only necessary to validate phosphorylation dependent staining and this portion of the protocol is dispensable when just staining for pRB. Ideally slides used for this validation step are consecutive sections of the same tissue such that one is mock dephosphorylated and stained with phosphospecific antibodies as described in Subheading 3.6 and later, and the other is phosphatase treated as described here before resuming the staining protocol in Subheading 3.6. In addition, we often use this validation step to quality control each lot of purchased phosphospecific antibodies, and once we are satisfied that detection is dependent on phosphorylation this step is omitted.

5. It is advisable to use the negative control slides, where primary antibody was omitted, to gauge staining and precise development times. Low background on the negative controls will allow longer color development without loss of specificity. Alternatively, higher staining on the negative controls may necessitate shortening the DAB incubation time.

Acknowledgments

The authors wish to thank the CIHR strategic training program in cancer research and technology transfer for fellowship support for CAI. FAD is the Wolfe Senior Research Fellow in Tumor Suppressor Genes at Western University. Research in the Dick lab is supported by the Canadian Institutes of Health Research and the Cancer Research Society.

References

1. Classon M, Harlow E (2002) The retinoblastoma tumour suppressor in development and cancer. Nat Rev Cancer 2:910–917

2. Dick FA, Rubin SM (2013) Molecular mechanisms underlying RB protein function. Nat Rev Mol Cell Biol 14(5):297–306

3. Dyson NJ (2016) RB1: a prototype tumor suppressor and an enigma. Genes Dev 30(13):1492–1502

4. Cecchini MJ, Ishak CA, Passos DT, Warner A, Palma DA, Howlett CJ, Driman DK, Dick FA (2015) Loss of the retinoblastoma tumor sup-

pressor correlates with improved outcome in patients with lung adenocarcinoma treated with surgery and chemotherapy. Hum Pathol 46(12):1922–1934

5. Zhao W, Huang CC, Otterson GA, Leon ME, Tang Y, Shilo K, Villalona MA (2012) Altered p16(INK4) and RB1 expressions are associated with poor prognosis in patients with nonsmall cell lung cancer. J Oncol 2012:957437. https://doi.org/10.1155/2012/957437

6. Ludovini V, Gregorc V, Pistola L, Mihaylova Z, Floriani I, Darwish S, Stracci F, Tofanetti FR, Ferraldeschi M, Di Carlo L, Ragusa M, Daddi G, Tonato M (2004) Vascular endothelial growth factor, p53, Rb, Bcl-2 expression and response to chemotherapy in advanced non-small cell lung cancer. Lung Cancer 46(1):77–85

7. Sherr CJ, Beach D, Shapiro GI (2015) Targeting CDK4 and CDK6: from discovery to therapy. Cancer Discov 6(4):353–367. https://doi.org/10.1158/2159-8290.CD-15-0894

8. Hewitson TD, Wigg B, Becker GJ (2010) Tissue preparation for histochemistry: fixation, embedding, and antigen retrieval for light microscopy. Methods Mol Biol 611: 3–18

9. Hirschi A, Cecchini M, Steinhardt RC, Schamber MR, Dick FA, Rubin SM (2010) An overlapping kinase and phosphatase docking site regulates activity of the retinoblastoma protein. Nat Struct Mol Biol 17(9): 1051–1057

10. Cecchini MJ, Dick FA (2011) The biochemical basis of CDK phosphorylation-independent regulation of E2F1 by the retinoblastoma protein. Biochem J 434(2):297–308

11. Francis SM, Bergsied J, Isaac CE, Coschi CH, Martens AL, Hojilla CV, Chakrabarti S, Dimattia GE, Khoka R, Wang JY, Dick FA (2009) A functional connection between pRB and transforming growth factor beta in growth inhibition and mammary gland development. Mol Cell Biol 29(16):4455–4466

Chapter 8

Immunohistochemical Detection of Retinoblastoma Protein Phosphorylation in Human Tumor Samples

Jaileene Pérez-Morales, Angel Núñez-Marrero, and Pedro G. Santiago-Cardona

Abstract

The retinoblastoma protein (pRb) is an important tumor suppressor and cell cycle repressor. pRb is a phosphoprotein whose function is regulated primarily at the level of phosphorylation, and therefore, detecting pRb's phosphorylation status in human tissue samples can be clinically informative. Unfortunately, detection of phosphorylated pRb residues can be technically challenging, as these residues can often be weak antigens. In this chapter, we describe an enhanced sensitivity immunohistochemistry protocol for the staining of phosphorylated serine 249 in pRb, in human lung tumor samples.

Key words Retinoblastoma protein, Tumor microarrays, Cell cycle control, Phosphorylation, Lung cancer, Immunohistochemistry

1 Introduction

The retinoblastoma protein (pRb) is an important tumor suppressor that acts as a cell cycle repressor, specifically controlling the G1–S transition of the cell cycle [1–5]. pRb is a phosphoprotein whose function is regulated primarily at the level of phosphorylation, its hyperphosphorylation being associated with a functionally repressed state [6–8]. Studying pRb's phosphorylation state is relevant both to the understanding of oncogenic mechanisms (as most human cancers exhibit hyperphosphorylated pRb), and also in a clinical setting, as pRb hyperphosphorylation can be a surrogate of pRb tumoral activity and therefore may have prognostic value.

Immunohistochemical staining for total pRb expression as well as for phosphorylation of several of its residues in human tumor samples can be clinically informative. In particular, phosphorylation of pRb in specific residues can be assessed by using commercially available phosphospecific pRb antibodies in immunohistochemical staining of human tumor samples. The study of pRb phosphorylation

Pedro G. Santiago-Cardona (ed.), *The Retinoblastoma Protein*, Methods in Molecular Biology, vol. 1726,
https://doi.org/10.1007/978-1-4939-7565-5_8, © Springer Science+Business Media, LLC 2018

in human tissues has been focused primordially on the phosphorylations that are known to be particularly disruptive of pRb's function as a cell cycle repressor. These phosphorylations usually occur in serine or threonine residues in pRb's pocket domain and in its C-terminal [9]. These phosphorylations are known to disrupt pRb's cell cycle repressive capacity by blocking pRb's capacity to bind and block the activities of the proliferation-related E2F transcription factors [9]. However, the paradigm of pRb function that is currently emerging is that of a multifunctional protein whose functions go beyond cell cycle control and that encompass other aspects of cellular physiology. In this context, noncanonical pRb phosphorylations (i.e., phosphorylations in other pRb domains that do not necessarily disrupt E2F interactions and cell cycle control) are emerging as phosphorylations of potential interest, both due to their potential clinical implications, as well as for their implications in the biochemical pathways related to pRb's antioncogenic function.

In this chapter, we explain the immunohistochemical staining of a pRb noncanonical phosphorylation in serine 249, in human lung tumor samples that were arranged as a tumor microarray. Phosphorylated residues can sometimes be weak antigens and therefore may present problems to their detection. Therefore, their detection may sometimes call for protocols with enhanced sensitivity. Here we describe specifically a protocol that uses the BioGenex Super Sensitive Link-Label IHC kit. The sensitivity of this kit relies on a secondary antibody to which multiple biotin residues have been conjugated in such a manner that the signal is amplified after streptavidin–horseradish peroxidase forms a complex with each biotin. This method is particularly suitable for antigens that give a weak signal using other immunohistochemical staining methods.

2   Materials

This protocol was optimized for formalin-fixed, paraffin-embedded (FFPE) tissues that were part of a commercially available lung cancer tumor microarray. However, you can also get your tissue slides prepared by your institutional histology services facility (*see* **Note 1**). It is therefore assumed that you have your tissues slides already available before starting this procedure.

2.1 Tissue Processing and Staining Reagents

1. Xylene (*see* **Note 2**).

2. Ethanol wash series. You need absolute (100%) ethanol, and then prepare 95%, 90%, 85%, 80% and 75% ethanol dilutions in distilled water (dH$_2$O).

3. Citrate antigen retrieval solution: Dissolve 1.92 g of trisodium citrate dehydrate and 0.74 g of EDTA in 800 ml of H$_2$O,

adjust pH to 6.2 with 1 N HCl, add 0.5 ml of Tween 20, and complete to final volume of 1 l. This solution can be stored at 4 °C for up to 6 months (*see* **Note 3**).

4. 1× PBS: dissolve 8 g NaCl, 0.2 g KCl, 1.44 g $Na_2HPO_4 \cdot 2$ H_2O, and 0.24 g of KH_2PO_4 in 800 ml of water. Adjust the pH to 7.2 with HCL, and add distilled water to complete the volume to 1 l. Keep at 4 °C.

5. 3% Hydrogen peroxide solution (*see* **Note 4**).

6. PAP Pen, this is used for drawing hydrophobic barriers around tissue slides.

7. Primary antibody: we optimized this protocol using a rabbit polyclonal antibody recognizing pRb phosphorylated in serine 249 purchased from Sigma-Aldrich (Anti-Phospho-Rb (S249), Cat. No. SAB 1305396-400 ml). We have tried both 1:50 and 1:100 dilutions with good results. Make your dilutions in 1× PBS. For 1:50, add 20 µl of antibody to 980 µl of PBS, and for a 1:100 dilution add 10 µl of antibody to 990 µl of 1× PBS.

8. Super Sensitive Link-Label IHC (BioGenex Cat. No. LP000-ULE). This is a kit that includes a biotin-labeled anti-rabbit secondary antibody. The kit also includes a streptavidin-conjugated horseradish peroxidase (HRP) (*see* **Note 5**).

9. Blocking solution: we use a blocking solution that is compatible with the Super Sensitive Link-Label IHC. This is a protein block sold by BioGenex (Cat. No. HK112-9K).

10. Diaminobenzidine (DAB). This is a substrate for the HRP, it produces a dark brown precipitate when oxidized by the HRP. We use the DAB solution provided by BioGenex (two-component kit, Cat. No. HK542-XAKE).

2.2 Additional Laboratory Equipment and Solutions

1. Conventional oven.

2. Humid chamber (*see* **Note 6**).

3. Standard cover glasses.

4. Mounting medium (*see* **Note 7**).

5. Standard slide racks and jars.

6. Microscope with camera, and suitable image capture software.

7. Pasteur or plastic pipettes.

8. Distilled water.

9. Lint-free tissue paper (e.g., Kimwipes or any other brand, provided it is lint-free).

10. Hot water bath.

3 Methods

1. Place the slides in a slide rack, and place them in an oven at 57 °C for 30 min. This will melt the paraffin and will facilitate the deparaffinization process.

2. Remove paraffin from tissues by submerging slides in their rack in xylene (or xylene substitute) for 30 min. Remember that this step should be performed inside a fume hood.

3. Hydrate the slides by subjecting them to ethanol washes as follows: 100% ethanol for 6 min, 95% ethanol for 3 min, 80% ethanol for 3 min, and 75% ethanol for 3 min. Complete hydration by submerging the slide in distilled H_2O for 1 min.

4. Place the slides flat in the humid chamber. From this point onward, avoid slides getting dry. In the subsequent steps, ensure that the tissue sections are completely soaked in the indicated solutions.

5. Rinse tissue sections on the slides with 1× PBS. You can add approximately 1 ml of PBS on top of the slide (using a Pasteur pipette), paying special attention that you are covering the entire slide surface and that all tissue sections are soaked in PBS. Do two washes of 5 min each.

6. Cover tissue sections with a layer of 3% hydrogen peroxide block to inactivate endogenous peroxidase activity. Incubate for 15 min.

7. Rinse tissue sections with 1× PBS, do two rinses of 5 min each.

8. Return the slides to a slide rack, and place the rack in a jar filled with the citrate antigen retrieval solution.

9. Perform the antigen retrieval step by submerging the jar (you need to cover the jar first) in a water bath that has been pre-heated to 95–99 °C. Leave the jar in the water bath for 40 min.

10. Remove the jar from the water bath and let it cool down to room temperature for 20–30 min.

11. Remove the slide rack from the jar, and submerge in distilled water for 2 min.

12. Remove slides from the rack, and place them flat in the humid chamber. Rinse tissue sections once with 1× PBS for 5 min.

13. Carefully dry the slides with a Kimwipes, only in the areas surrounding the tissues (avoid damaging the tissue sections!). After drying the glass surrounding the tissue sections, use the PAP pen to make a hydrophobic circle surrounding the tissue section. Again, be careful not to damage the tissues.

14. Perform the blocking step by adding enough volume of the blocking solution to cover the tissue section. Incubate at room temperature for 1 h inside the humid chamber.

15. Carefully remove the excess of blocking solution and dry the slides with a Kimwipes. Avoid damaging the tissue sections in this step. You can achieve this by tilting the slide sideways and removing the solution from the edge of the slide. Do not rinse after removing the blocking solution.

16. Incubate in the primary antibody by adding a drop of antibody solution to each tissue section. At this step, the slides should be in the humid chamber. Incubate overnight (12–18 h) at 4–8 °C (*see* **Note 8**). Remember to perform negative control sections in which the primary antibody is omitted. These are done by incubating tissues in 1× PBS instead of antibody solution.

17. Remove the primary antibody and rinse the slides a total of three washes, 5 min each (*see* **Note 9**). Remove excess PBS with a Kimwipes, but remember that tissue sections must never get dry.

18. Incubate in secondary antibody by covering the tissue sections with enough solution. Incubation should be in the humid chamber at room temperature for 30 min.

19. Remove the secondary antibody solution and wash the slides three times with 1× PBS, 5 min each wash. After the last wash, remove excess liquid with a Kimwipes.

20. Add the streptavidin–HRP mix to each tissue section, and incubate in the humid chamber for 30 min at room temperature.

21. Remove the streptavidin–HRP mix and wash the slides with 1× PBS three times, 5 min each wash. Remove excess PBS after last wash.

22. Prepare the DAB solution following manufacturer's directions, and add a drop of solution to each tissue section. Incubate for a maximum of 2 min. When we use the antibody dilutions of 1:50 or 1:100, we have noticed that the optimal signal developing time is around 1 min, but you must empirically determine the optimal incubation time (*see* **Note 10**).

23. Stop the DAB reaction by placing the slides in their rack and submerging them in a jar with distilled water. Leave the slides in their rack under running tap water for 5 min, being careful that the water does not directly touch the tissue sections.

24. Dehydrate the slides with ethanol baths as follows: 85%, 90%, 95%, and absolute (100%) ethanol, 2 min in each bath.

25. Incubate the slides in xylene for 2 min.

26. Drain the xylene from the slides and dry them in an oven at 37 °C for 30 min.

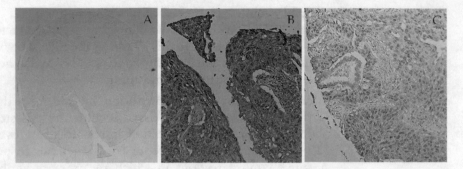

Fig. 1 Lung tumor tissue sections immunohistochemically stained using an anti Rb phosphoSer249 antibody. (**a**) negative control in which the primary antibody was omitted. (**b**) primary antibody at a 1:50 dilution. (**c**) primary antibody at a 1:100 dilution. Notice the high intensity of the staining when using the antibody diluted at 1:50 (**b**). The intense staining makes it difficult to appreciate the expected pRb nuclear localization. For that reason, we determined 1:100 as the optimal dilution for this antibody (**c**), as this dilution allows for a better definition of stained nuclei

27. Add 2–3 drops of mounting media on top of each tissue section and carefully place a coverslip on top of the section, avoiding the formation of air bubbles inside the preparation. Wipe excess mounting media from the edges using a Kimwipes (*see* **Note 11**).

28. Analyze slides under a light microscope. A representative staining with the Rb anti-phospho (S249) can be seen in Fig. 1. A clearly defined nuclear staining can be discerned when we use the 1:100 primary antibody dilution. It is recommended that you enlist a pathologist to help you with the scoring. We usually use a two-dimensional scoring system that measures intensity of staining (0, +1, +2, +3) as well as the % of stained cells in a visual field.

4 Notes

1. Be sure that thickness of tissue sections is 4–10 μm. It is also important that the tissue is intact without breaks or folds, as these usually result in staining artifacts.

2. Steps using solvents like xylene must be performed inside a fume hood, and xylene waste must be discarded according to biohazards regulations. Regular xylene can be used, but we use ThermoFisher Shandon Xylene Substitute (Cat. No. 9990505) as it is safer than regular xylene. It has a similar evaporation rate to regular xylene, but it is less sensitizing to skin, and is safer than xylene regarding airborne exposure. Still, we recommend, if possible to handle this reagent within a fume hood.

3. We recommend that you include EDTA in the antigen retrieval buffer when using phosphospecific antibodies. This inhibits endogenous phosphatase activity, therefore enhancing the staining.

4. We use BioGenex Hydrogen Peroxide block (Cat. No. HK111-50K), but standard hydrogen peroxide diluted to 3% will work well. This solution blocks endogenous peroxidase activity, a step that is crucial when using secondary antibodies conjugated to horseradish peroxidase (HRP). Omitting this step will result in high background resulting from the activity of endogenous peroxidases on the DAB substrate. Liver, kidney, and red blood cells are particularly high in endogenous peroxidase activity, but you should nevertheless include this step when processing other tissues as well.

5. The kit's secondary antibody has multiple biotin residues, so the advantage of this kit is its improved sensitivity to weak antigens (such as a phosphospecific antigen), due to signal amplification. Strictly follow the manufacturer's instructions when preparing the solution of this antibody.

6. All incubations should be carried out in a humidified chamber to avoid drying of the tissues. Drying of the tissue may lead to nonspecific binding of the antibody and high background. You do not need to buy a commercially available humid chamber, you can build your own from inexpensive components. Any plastic container with a lid that produces a tight seal will be adequate. You can use an inverted pipette tip case cover as a platform to place your slides. For humidity, paper towels soaked in PBS will be sufficient.

7. You can prepare your own mounting medium, but most commercially available mediums will work well. The important thing to keep in mind is that the mounting medium of choice will be determined by the nature and solubility of the precipitate that will be formed by the action of the enzyme conjugated to the secondary antibody. In this protocol, we use the diaminobenzidine (DAB) substrate for the horseradish peroxidase enzyme conjugated to the secondary antibody. Be sure that your mounting medium is compatible with this system.

8. Prolonged incubations at low temperatures can dry your slides. For this incubation, be sure that the humid chamber has plenty of PBS. Do not allow the antibody solution to overflood and pass to the adjacent sections. Dilution of the primary antibody is one of the parameters that you can modify should you need to do some troubleshooting to improve the signal. If you are troubled by high background, try diluting the primary antibody more or blocking for a longer time.

9. Thoroughly wash the slides to avoid background; also the slides should never be left to dry.

10. Set up a timer; try not to go beyond 2 min. This step will produce a dark brown precipitate as the HRP acts on the DAB substrate. Too long a development time can produce very high background. It may be advisable to monitor the darkening of the staining by visualizing the dark precipitate under a light microscope. You may want to add an additional hematoxylin and eosin counterstaining step after this step.

11. Properly sealed slides can last indefinitely stored at room temperature inside a slide box.

References

1. Harbour JW, Dean DC (2000) Rb function in cell-cycle regulation and apoptosis. Nat Cell Biol 2(4):E65–E67

2. Dyson N (1998) The regulation of E2F by pRB-family proteins. Genes Dev 12:2245–2262

3. Ross JF, Liu X, Dynlacht BD (1999) Mechanism of transcriptional repression of E2F by the retinoblastoma tumor suppressor protein. Mol Cell 3:195–205

4. Thomas DM, Carty SA, Piscopo DM, Lee J-S, Wang W-F et al (2001) The retinoblastoma protein acts as a transcriptional coactivator required for osteogenic differentiation. Mol Cell 8:303–316

5. Thomas DM, Yang H-S, Alexander K, Hinds PW (2003) Role of the retinoblastoma protein in differentiation and senescence. Cancer Biol Ther 2:2–8

6. Rubin SM (2013) Deciphering the retinoblastoma protein phosphorylation code. Trends Biochem Sci 38(1):12–19

7. Lundberg AS, Weinberg RA (1998) Functional inactivation of the retinoblastoma protein requires sequential modification by at least two distinct cyclin-cdk complexes. Mol Cell Biol 18(2):753–761

8. Buchkovich K, Duffy LA, Harlow E (1989) The retinoblastoma protein is phosphorylated during specific phases of the cell cycle. Cell 58(6):1097–1105

9. Burke JR, Liban TJ, Restrepo T, Lee HW, Rubin SM (2014) Multiple mechanisms for E2F binding inhibition by phosphorylation of the retinoblastoma protein C-terminal domain. J Mol Biol 426(1):245–255

Chapter 9

Detection of CCND1 Locus Amplification by Fluorescence In Situ Hybridization

Margit Balázs, Viktória Koroknai, István Szász, and Szilvia Ecsedi

Abstract

It is well known that chromosomal aberrations of tumors are associated with the initiation and progression of malignancy. Fluorescence in situ hybridization (FISH) is a powerful, rapid method to detect chromosome copy number and structural alterations in tissue sections, chromosome, or interphase cellular preparations via hybridization of complementary probe sequences. The technique is based on the complementary nature of DNA double strands, which allows fluorescently labeled DNA probes to be used as probes to label the complementary sequences of target cells, chromosomes, and tissues. FISH technique has many applications, including basic gene mapping, used in pathological diagnosis to detect chromosome and gene copy number aberrations, translocations, microdeletions, and duplications. For the recognition of gene amplifications and deletions, locus-specific probes that are collections of one or a few cloned DNA sequences are routinely used. Multiplex-FISH (M-FISH) technique visualizes all chromosomes with different colors using spectrally distinct fluorophores for each chromosome in one experiment to detect numerical and structural alterations of chromosomes obtained from tumor cells. Recently many of the gene-specific probes are commercially available.

Key words Fluorescence in situ hybridization, DNA probes, Gene amplification in interphase cells, CCND1 copy number alteration

1 Introduction

1.1 CCND1 Locus Amplification and Its Role in Cancer Etiology and Diagnostics

The Cyclin D1 (CCND1) proto-oncogene has a major role in the regulation of the cell cycle by encoding the regulatory subunit of the enzyme that phosphorylates and inactivates the retinoblastoma protein (pRb) [1, 2]. Inactivation of pRb leads to the release of E2F transcription factors, causing the progression from the G1 to the S phase of the cell cycle [3]. Aberration in this regulatory process of the cell cycle occurs frequently in human cancer, and the alteration of cyclin D1 is one of the most commonly observed events [1, 4].

The CCND1 locus is located at the 11q13 chromosomal region that is a frequently amplified in several types of human tumors including breast cancer, melanoma, head and neck squamous cell carcinoma or laryngeal squamous cell carcinoma [5–10]. Moreover,

Pedro G. Santiago-Cardona (ed.), *The Retinoblastoma Protein*, Methods in Molecular Biology, vol. 1726,
https://doi.org/10.1007/978-1-4939-7565-5_9, © Springer Science+Business Media, LLC 2018

the amplification of the CCND1 gene is usually correlated with clinicopathological parameters indicating its role in tumor development [6, 11, 12]. A recent study revealed that amplified CCND1 may offer a direct target for molecular therapy in advanced gastric cancer [13].

The analysis of CCND1 copy number using FISH technique provides the opportunity to calculate copy number index (CNI), which can be a predictive marker in several tumor types including melanoma. Furthermore, a diagnostic melanoma FISH test, performed with a panel of four probes including CCND1 gene, is a useful tool to distinguish between benign and malignant melanocytic neoplasms [14]. Moreover, FISH results confirmed that among these four genetic loci the CCND1 seems to be the most specific probe in the diagnosis of melanoma [15]. It has been proved that the FISH technique is crucial in the detection of CCND1 amplification whose copy number alteration is considered as candidate driver for malignant tumors.

1.2 Technical Aspects of FISH

The schematic illustration of the FISH technique is summarized on Fig. 1. Double stranded target DNA (tissue section, interphase cells, chromosomes preparations) and fluorescently labeled DNA probes are denatured at 70–75 °C (usually for 3–5 min) and incubated together under certain conditions (usually at 37–42 °C depending on the probe, overnight). This condition permits bindings of the labeled DNA probes to the complementary target sequences. The fluorescently labeled probe that hybridizes to the DNA in the cell nucleus appears as a distinct fluorescent dot. The number of fluorescent signals can be evaluated using a fluorescent microscope or image system.

1.3 Major Classes of DNA-Specific Probes

1.3.1 Centromere-Specific Probes

These probes target the centromeric regions of chromosomes which contain tandemly repeated short sequences as compact clusters (sometimes spanning a few megabases) (Fig. 2). The different repeats are labeled as a, b, and c in Fig. 2. The chromosome arms contain mixtures of unique and interspersed sequences [16]. Figure 3 shows examples of FISH using centromere-specific probes (a), combination of centromeric and locus-specific probes and whole chromosome painting probes (c and d). Centromere-specific probes are alpha repetitive sequences and are frequently used in combination with locus (gene)-specific probes (discussed below) in order to distinguish between aneuploidy and gene amplifications (Fig. 3a).

1.3.2 Locus- and Gene-Specific Probes

These probes are very useful for the rapid identification of a large number of chromosome segment aberrations. They are used to detect gene amplifications, deletions, and various rearrangements frequently observed in different tumors and other diseases (Fig. 3b).

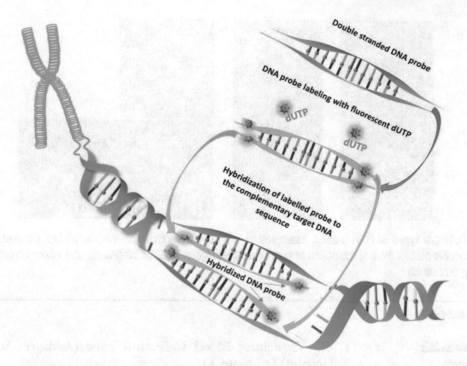

Fig. 1 Schematic drawing of fluorescence in situ hybridization. Double stranded DNA probes and target DNA are denatured in order to become accessible during renaturation

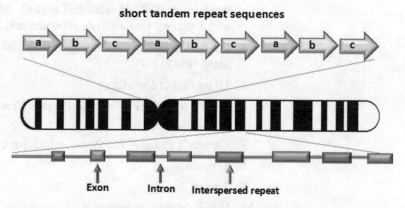

Fig. 2 Overview of the DNA sequence structure of human chromosomes. The centromeric regions contains tandemly repeated sequences, the different repeats are labelled with **a**, **b**, and **c**

1.3.3 Whole Chromosome (Painting) Probes

These types of probes can be used only on chromosome spreads and bind along the length of a given chromosome. Using multiple fluorescent dyes, they make it possible to label each chromosome with a different label, resulting in a spectral karyotype. The major advantage of these types of probes is their capacity to detect chromosomal translocations (Fig. 3c, d).

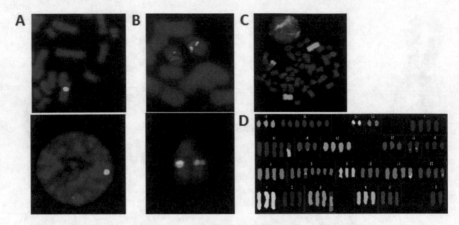

Fig. 3 Different types of FISH probes. Examples of FISH using centromere-specific probes (**a**), locus- and genes-pecific probes (**b**), a combination of centromeric and locus-specific probes (**c**), and whole chromosome painting probes (**d**)

2   Materials

2.1   Materials for Sample Preparation

1. BD Vacutainer® Blood Collection Tube (Additive: Sodium Heparin) (*see* **Note 1**).

2. Heparinized blood (3–5 ml).

3. Peripheral blood karyotyping medium: RPMI 1640 medium containing 20% of fetal calf serum, 300 μg/ml L-glutamine, and 1 μg/ml penicillin/streptomycin.

4. 0.1 ml Gibco® Phytohemagglutinin, M form (mitogen to stimulate cells).

5. 10 μg/ml colcemid.

6. 68–75 mM KCl in distilled water (freshly prepared hypotonic solution, 100 ml).

7. Carnoy's fixative: methanol–glacial acetic acid (3:1).

8. Trypsin.

9. Tween 20.

10. Ethyl alcohol, anhydrous.

11. Formaldehyde (37%).

12. 2 M magnesium chloride ($MgCl_2$).

13. Methyl alcohol, anhydrous.

14. Pepsin.

15. 1× (or 0.01 M) Phosphate Buffered Saline (PBS). To prepare, dissolve 8 g NaCl, 0.2 g KCl, 1.44 g $Na_2HPO_4 \cdot 2H_2O$, and 0.24 g of KH_2PO_4 in 800 ml of water. Adjust the pH to 7.2 with HCl, and add distilled water to complete the volume to 1 l.

16. 1× RNase.

17. 20× SSC: 175.3 g NaCl; 88.2 g of sodium citrate dissolved in distilled H_2O (dH_2O) final volume is 1 l; adjust the pH to 7.0 with 1 M HCl; autoclave the solution and store at room temperature.

18. 1 M sodium isothiocyanate (NaSCN).

19. Xylene, 100%.

20. ddH_2O.

21. Graded ethyl alcohol: dilute with ddH_2O to 70%, 85%, 90%. You need also 100% ethanol.

22. 70% Formamide/2× SSC: 10 ml 20× SSC, 20 ml dH_2O, 70 ml deionized formamide, adjust to pH 7.0 with HCl, aliquot and store at −20 °C.

23. 4× SSC/Tween 20: 100 ml 20× SSC, 400 ml H_2O, 0.5% Tween 20, keep at room temperature.

24. Pepsin, 10% stock solution: Dissolve 100 mg/ml pepsin in dH_2O, make 50 μl aliquots and store at −20 °C.

25. Pepsin, working solution: always make the solution fresh before the slide treatment step, place 5–30 μl pepsin into 37 °C prewarmed diluted HCl (99 ml dH_2O + 1 ml 1 N HCl). (Avoid repeated thawing and usage of pepsin over time will weaken catalytic activity.)

26. $PBS/MgCl_2$: 25 ml of 2 M $MgCl_2$ in 950 ml 1× PBS.

27. $Formaldehyde/PBS/MgCl_2$: 2.7 ml 37% formaldehyde 100 ml $PBS/MgCl_2$.

2.2 Fluorescence In Situ Hybridization

2.2.1 DNA Labeling with Nick Translation

1. 10× A4 dNTP mix: prepare this by mixing the following components:

   – 5 μl of 10 mM dATP, 5 μl of 10 mM dCTP, 5 μl of 10 mM dGTP (final concentration is 200 μM, 10×).

   – 125 μl 1 M Tris–HCl, pH 7.2 (final 500 μM, 10×).

   – 12.5 μl 1 M $MgCl_2$ (final 200 μM, 10×).

   – 1.7 μl 14.7 M mercaptoethanol (100 mM, 10×).

   – 0.5 μl 50 mg/ml BSA (final 100 μg/ml, 10×).

   – 95.3 μl dH_2O to reach a final volume of 250 μl.

   – Aliquot and store at −20 °C in screw cap tubes.

2. 25 nm fluorescently labeled dUTP (10×).

3. 10 mM unlabeled dUTP.

4. DNA Polymerase I.

5. DNA Polymerase/DNase I: 10× Enzyme ("fast enzyme") Mix. This is from the BioNick kit (GIBCO, Thermo Fisher Scientific).

6. DNA Pol-1/DNase I (alternative of the 10× enzyme mix). This is a "slow enzyme" mix from Thermo Fisher Scientific (Catalog No. 18162-016).

7. Agarose for gel electrophoresis.

2.2.2 Hybridization and Detection

1. It is very convenient to perform the FISH using a programmable Slide Denaturation and Hybridization System (e.g., Leica) such as the one shown in Fig. 4 (http://www.leicabio-systems.com/ihc-ish-fish/ish-probes-molecular-pathology/kreatech-fish-probes/equipment/thermobriter/). Other companies produce alternative hybridization systems for FISH protocols, for example the Slide Moat™ by Boekel Scientific, which provides excellent temperature uniformity and stability, with a capacity for 30 slides. If no hybridization system is available, the procedure can be performed using a water bath in which the denaturation can be performed in a jar containing the denaturation solution described below.

2. 20× SSC, prepared as described in Subheading 2.1.

3. Denaturation Solution: 70% Formamide/2× SSC, pH 7.0. To prepare, mix 4 ml 20× SSC, 8 ml ddH$_2$O, 28 ml Formamide, 40 ml final volume. Prepare fresh for each assay on the day of use in a conical 50 ml centrifuge tube, and adjust pH to 7.0 with 6 N HCl. This solution is not needed when using a programmable Slide Denaturation and Hybridization System. Use only when denaturation is performed in a water bath.

4. Post-Hybridization Wash Solution: 50% formamide/2× SSC, pH 7.0. Prepare by mixing 4 ml 20× SSC, 16 ml distilled water, 20 ml formamide, 40 ml final volume. The solution can be stored at 4 °C for 1 week.

5. Hybridization buffer: 55% formamide (high purity), 10% dextran sulfate (weight/volume), 0.1% Tween 20, 1× SSC and adjust the pH to 7.0.

6. Graded ethyl alcohol series (EtOH): 100%, and diluted with ddH$_2$O to 70%, 85%, 100% in Coplin jars, keep on ice.

7. Probe mix: 10 μl for each slide containing 10–20 ng for centromeric and 40 ng for cosmid probes in hybridization buffer (55% formamide, 1× SSC/10% dextran sulfate, 1 μg unlabeled sonicated Cot1 DNA (200–500 bp), leave on ice until use.

8. DAPI or propidium iodide.

9. Vectashield Mounting Medium.

10. Fluorescence microscope equipped with selective filters for the detection of FITC, SpectrumGreen, SpectrumOrange, and DAPI. You also need an accompanying appropriate digital imaging analysis system for detection and generation of three-color images.

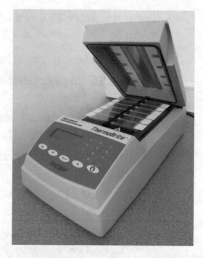

Fig. 4 ThermoBrite apparatus recommended for FISH. Complete specifications for this can be found at http://www.leicabiosystems.com/ihc-ish-fish/ish-probes-molecular-pathology/kreatech-fish-probes/equipment/thermobriter/

2.3 General Labware and Equipment

1. Sterile T25 flasks.

2. Falcon tubes (15 and 50 ml).

3. Water baths (37 °C, 45 °C).

4. Glass pipettes.

5. Centrifuge.

6. Clean superfrost microscopic slides (wash in absolute ethanol overnight) and slide boxes.

7. Slide storage boxes.

8. CO_2 incubator.

9. Coplin jars.

10. Rotating shaker.

11. Coverslips 22×22 mm.

12. Rubber cement.

3 Methods

3.1 Preparation of Metaphase Chromosomes from Peripheral Blood

The peripheral blood of a healthy individual is the most frequently used tissue to obtain normal chromosome preparation to test the specificity of hybridization. The quality of metaphase chromosomes is very important, especially in routine diagnostics. All different FISH probes can be used to detect alterations on metaphase chromosomes, while chromosome painting probes are not informative to detect abnormalities in interphase nuclei. The most frequently used protocol to prepare chromosomes from white blood cells is the stimulation of cells with 10 µg/ml phytohemagglutinin.

For different cell types and specific methods, detailed methods are given by Saunders et al. [17].

1. Collect blood into a heparinized vacutainer tube.

2. Add 10 ml peripheral blood karyotyping medium to each sterile T25 flask.

3. Add 0.75 ml blood into each flask, loose the caps and incubate in a CO_2 incubator for 72 h.

4. Add 0.1 µg/ml colcemid to each flask, mix well and incubate for 20 min.

5. After 20 min, transfer flask contents into a 15 ml centrifuge tube and spin down at $300 \times g$ for 10 min.

6. Remove supernatant only leave 0.5 ml above the cell pellet and suspend cells carefully.

7. Add 2 ml of prewarmed (37 °C) hypotonic solution (KCl) drop-by-drop to the cell pellet while agitating the cell suspension gently.

8. Add an additional 8 ml hypotonic solution, for a final volume of 10 ml and mix well.

9. Incubate the cells for 15 min at 37 °C, mix in each 5 min.

10. Add a few drops of the methanol–acetic acid fixative, recap the tube and invert to mix.

11. Centrifuge cell suspension and remove supernatant similarly as in **step 6**.

12. Add ice-cold fixative, drop by drop the first 2 ml while agitating very gently, add finally 10 ml fixative and leave at room temperature for 10–15 min.

13. Centrifuge cells and remove supernatant similarly as in **step 6**.

14. Repeat the fixation at least three more times.

15. After the last centrifugation, remove supernatant and suspend the cells in a small volume of fixative (maximum 1 ml).

16. Slide must be very clean. Wipe slides dry with a lint-free tissue. Drop small drops of cell suspension onto slide surface with a Pasteur pipet and allow it to spread. Dropping one drop of fixative onto the cell suspension once it has started to dry may be done to increase the spreading of the chromosomes (*see* **Note 2**).

17. Leave the slides to dry overnight at room temperature.

18. It is possible to keep slides in boxes at −20 °C for a few years in a sealed plastic bag.

19. Always avoid water condensation on the glass slides! (*see* **Note 3**).

3.2 Chromosome Preparation from Adherent Cells

1. Grow cells to reach 80% of confluency (logarithmic phase), at that point add 10 µl/ml of colcemid to the cell culture (at least 2×10^6 cells are recommended).

2. Incubate cells at 37 °C (5% CO_2 incubator) for 45 min. Transfer media from cells into a sterile tube. Set it aside since it will be needed later.

3. Gently wash the cells in the flask by adding 2 ml of RPMI into the flask. Swirl buffer and then remove it by Pasteur pipette. Discard.

4. Add 1 ml trypsin (0.05–0.25% in Hank's Buffered Salt Solution, calcium- and magnesium-free, depending on cell types), be sure that it covers the entire surface of the flask. Once the majority of cells have detached the bottom of the flask (usually it is 2 min, do not leave it longer), pipette back the media onto the cells from the sterile tube to stop the trypsin.

5. Transfer the cell suspension in 10 ml aliquots into 15 ml sterile tubes. Centrifuge at $300 \times g$ for 10 min. Remove supernatant and resuspend the cell pellet leaving 0.5 ml supernatant above the pellet.

6. From this step follow the protocol of the metaphase chromosome preparation from peripheral blood from **step 7** (Subheading 3.1).

3.3 Preparation of Tumor Imprints from Fresh and Frozen Tissues

Tumor imprint preparations are very useful especially for small tumors and are widely used samples for FISH analysis [18]. The natural propensity of tumor cells to adhere to a microscopic glass slide has been successfully used in touch imprint FISH.

1. Cut small piece from fresh or frozen tumor tissue and touch them very gently to a superfrost microscopic glass slide using sterile forceps.

2. Fixation of the tissue imprint: put the slides into a cold Coplin jar containing fixative (methanol–glacial acetic acid, 3:1), leave the slides in the jar for 10 min (*see* **Note 4**).

3. Remove the slides from the jar and let them dry at room temperature.

4. Collect the slides into a microscope slide box, seal in a plastic bag and keep at −20 °C until used for FISH analysis. Always avoid water condensation on the glass slides.

3.4 Frozen and Paraffin-Embedded Tissue Sections: Pretreatment Before FISH [19]

3.4.1 Pretreatment Protocol for Frozen Sections Only

1. Cut 5 μm sections from frozen tissue block and place on silanized slide.

2. Thaw slides at room temperature and equilibrate in 2× SSC for 5–10 min.

3. Place slides in diluted pepsin suspension containing 5–30 μl pepsin for 2–5 min. This is a critical step, its optimization depends on tissue age and the amount of stromal components.

4. Wash two times in PBS at RT, 5 min each.

5. Wash once in PBS/MgCl$_2$ at RT, for 5 min.

6. Wash in Formaldehyde/PBS/MgCl$_2$ for 10 min.

7. Wash in PBS for 5 min.

8. Dehydrate in 70%, 85%, and 100% ethanol for 3 min each and air-dry.

9. Fix in Carnoy's fixative for 5 min and leave to dry at room temperature.

3.4.2 Pretreatment Protocol for Formalin-Fixed, Paraffin-Embedded Tissue Sections Only

1. Tissues are sectioned using a microtome, optimal for FISH a 5 μm section.

2. Place slides with paraffin tissue sections into 100% xylene for 5 min, change xylene and repeat this step for another 5 min.

3. Rehydrate the tissue for 5 min each in 100% EtOH, 90% EtOH, and 70% EtOH (at room temperature).

4. Wash in 4× SSC/Tween 20 at RT for 30 min, use a rotating shaker.

5. For formalin-fixed slides, place in Coplin jar with 1 M NaSCN at room temperature and keep there overnight. Wear gloves when handling NaSCN!

6. Wash slides in distilled water for 5 min.

3.4.3 Pepsin Treatment and Fixation (For Both Paraffin-Embedded and Frozen Sections)

1. After the pretreatment steps above, place slides in diluted pepsin suspension containing 5–30 μl pepsin for fresh material and 20–500 μl pepsin for formalin fixed material for 2–5 min. (Critical step! *see* **Note 5**.)

2. Wash slides in PBS two times at RT, 5 min each.

3. Wash slides in PBS/MgCl$_2$ once at RT, for 5 min.

4. Wash slides in formaldehyde/PBS/MgCl$_2$ for 10 min.

5. Wash slides in PBS for 5 min.

6. Dehydrate in 70%, 90%, and 100% ethanol for 3 min each and air-dry.

3.5 FISH with Fluorescently Labeled DNA Probes

A wide variety of DNA probes can be used for FISH. DNA-specific probes can be prepared from different cloning vectors (BACs, YACs, PACs, cosmids, P1 clones). Table 1 summarizes the host, the structure, and the size of inserts for the different vectors [20].

Table 1
Examples for cloning vectors commonly used for FISH

Vector	Host	Structure	Insert size (kb)
Cosmids	*E. coli*	Circ. plasmid	35/45
P1 clones	*E. coli*	Circ. plasmid	70/100
BACs	*E. coli*	Circ. plasmid	Up to 300
PACs	*E. coli*	Circ. plasmid	100/300
YACs	*Saccharomyces cerevisiae*	Linear chromosomes	100/2000

Abbreviations: *BACs* bacterial artificial chromosomes, *PACs* P1 derived chromosomes, *YACs* yeast artificial chromosomes, *E. coli Escherichia coli*, *Circ. plasmid* circular plasmid [20]

After harvesting and lysing the host cells, the cloned DNA is purified from the host chromosomal DNA and cellular material using commercial kits (Qiagene, Thermo Fisher Scientific, Invitrogen). Bacterial cells containing the clone of interest are usually grown in media that selects for the clone by use of an antibiotic, or in the case of yeast, in media which lacks a particular nutrient. Detailed description for growing bacteria and for isolating DNA are described by Garimberti E and Tosi S [20]. In order to label the DNA fluorescently, the most frequently used protocol is nick translation (*see* **Note 6**). The procedure allows the incorporation of fluorescently labelled dUTPs. A wide range of fluorescent dyes are available for labeling. The most frequently used are: fluorescein isothiocyanate (FITC) and different cyanine fluorophores. A wide range of fluorescently labeled nucleotides are available from different companies (e.g., Thermo Fisher Scientific, MoBiTec, and PromoKine). The easiest way to perform nick translation is to use commercial kits, such as the ones available from vendors such as Enzo, GIBCO, Abbott Molecular, and Roche Ltd. Below is the modification of a nick translation protocol for plasmid or cosmid probes (adapted from Fred Waldman's Laboratory UCSF).

3.5.1 Nick Translation Reaction

When using the DNA Polymerase/DNase I: 10× Enzyme ("fast enzyme") mix, if this enzyme cuts the DNA too small, try varying the amount and/or time of incubation. The standard concentration for fresh DNA is 3 μl of 10× Enzyme mix for 60 min. Incorporation decreases appreciably below 2 μl DNA or with less than 40 min reactions. If the mix still cuts too small, with these minimum amounts, try the "slow" enzyme mix described below, or a mixture of the two. We attempt to freeze down one lot of 10× Enzyme with known characteristics to be used for several months.

If you decide to use the DNA Pol-1/DNase I (alternative of the 10× enzyme mix) or "slow enzyme" mix, this enzyme is less active than the 10× Enzyme mix from the BioNick kit. If it is necessary to use this, try for 60 min using 5 µl first, and adjust conditions as needed to get to optimal size of probes.

Preparation the reaction mixture for nick translation using fluorescently labeled dUTP as follows:

1. For each labeling reaction, on ice, prepare a tube containing the reagents for 50 µl nick translation reaction (keep all reagents on ice).

Reagents	Volume (µl)
10× fluorescently labeled-dUTP	5
10× A4 dNTP	5
10 mM unlabeled dUTP	1
DNA polymerase I (BioNick 10× enzyme mix)	1
DNA pol/DNAse (additional)	2.5–5
DNA (1 µg, the volume depends on the DNA probe concentration)	
ddH$_2$O (to complete 50 µl)	
Total reaction volume	50

2. Incubate reaction mixtures for 60 min at 15 °C (prepare in advance using ice bucket, water and ice, *see* **Note 7**).

3. Stop reaction by heating at 70 °C for 15 min.

4. Run 3–5 µl of probe on 1% agarose gel to check size. Product should run as a smear ranging from 0.3 to 2.3 kb.

5. Store probes at −20 °C.

3.5.2 Commercially Available Probes

Recently, mainly fluorescently labeled probes are available which are labeled with different fluorescent dyes. These are shown in Table 2. It is important that during the hybridization you must follow the steps as it is suggested by the supplier (*see* **Note 8**).

3.5.3 Fluorescence In Situ Hybridization

The FISH protocol described below is for cell lines and frozen tumor imprint preparations using the programmable slide warmer.

1. Wash slides in a Coplin jar in 2× SSC for 5 min.

2. Dehydrate slides through an alcohol series in 70%, 85%, 100% in Coplin jars (2 min each).

3. Allow slides to air-dry for at least 5 min.

4. Place slides on the programmable slide warmer (e.g., ThermoBrite). Using the temperature control, adjust the

Table 2
Types of CCND1 FISH probes available commercially

Empire genomics	For detection of	Size of the labeled probe
CCND1 FISH probe	Gene amplification	340 kb
CCND1 break apart FISH probe	Gene rearrangement	508 kb/727 kb
CCND1/IGH FISH probe	CCND1/IGH gene fusions	CCND1 340 kb/ IGH 1497 kb
Abnova		
CCND1/CEN11q FISH probe	Gene amplification/centromere copy number	162 kb
ZytoVysion		
CCND1 dual color break apart probe	Translocations of 11q13.3 harboring the CCND1 gene	635 kb to centromere/580 kb telomere
CCND1/CEN 11 dual color probe	Gene amplification/centromere copy number	825 kb
CCND1/IGH dual color dual fusion probe	CCND1/IGH gene fusions	1.5 Mb/1.5 Mb

denaturing temperature to 70–73 °C for 3–5 min (depending on the sample, it should be determined for each sample type). This instrument can hold 12 slides. It is important to note that when using a programmable Slide Denaturation and Hybridization System, there is no need to use the denaturation solution (70% formamide/2× SSC). In case no hybridization system is available, denaturation can be performed using a water bath. In that case, a jar with the denaturation solution should be placed into the water bath before turning the temperature to 70 °C. When the denaturing solution reaches this temperature, the slide should be denatured for 3–5 min and then dehydrated in the ethanol series at room temperature, followed by air drying. The probe mix should be applied after the slide is completely dry.

5. Adjust the renaturation temperature to 12–16 h.

6. Add 10 μl probe mix to each slide and cover with a 22 × 22 mm coverslip carefully, avoiding air bubbles and seal the coverslip with rubber cement.

7. Close the lid of the ThermoBrite instrument. It maintains uniform temperature across all slide positions.

8. After the renaturation step gently remove the rubber cement solution avoiding the movement of the coverslip that can result in the damage of chromosomes and cell nuclei.

9. Wash the slides in a Coplin jar containing 2× SSC to remove the coverslip, shaking the slides can speed up this step.

10. To remove the unbound or nonspecifically bound probe fragments, wash the slides in Post-Hybridization Wash Solution two times, once in 2× SSC and once in 0.1 SSC for 10 min each at 45 °C.

11. Place 15 μl of DAPI in a Vectashield mounting medium on each slide, cover with coverslip.

3.5.4 Evaluation
of Fluorescence In Situ
Hybridization Results

Specimens on slides are typically mounted in an antifade medium containing DNA counterstain such as DAPI (blue emitting dye excited at 360 nm) or propidium iodide (a red emitting dye excited between 480 and 550 nm). The microscope should be equipped with appropriate filter sets (excitation and emission filters) in order to view the fluorophores. During the last two decades, different image systems were developed for the accurate counting of FISH signals and to improve the image analysis of FISH images. In our laboratory, we use Zeiss microscope equipped with selective filters for the detection of FITC, SpectrumGreen, SpectrumOrange, and DAPI. Approximately 200–500 nuclei and/or 10 metaphases are scored for each hybridization. Three-color images are captured using a digital imaging analysis system (ISIS, Metasystems GmbH, Althussheim, Germany). Figure 5 shows a typical result of a FISH experiment with centromeric 11 (green signals) and CCND1 specific (red signals).

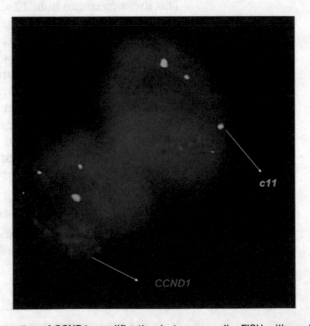

Fig. 5 Detection of CCND1 amplification in tumour cells. FISH with centromeric 11 (green signals) and CCND1 specific (red signals)

4   Notes

1. Note that anticoagulants such as EDTA cannot be used to culture blood cells because it is toxic for white blood cells.

2. It is possible to drop two drops of cells on one slide, but to obtain optimal spreading of chromosomes better to start only with one drop/slide. A method for improving metaphase chromosome spreading was tested by Deng W et al.; the authors provide very useful information for this step [21]. The quality and the concentration of cells and chromosomes can be checked under phase contrast after dropping the fixed cell suspension. The aim is to obtain pale grey chromosomes and nuclei free of cytoplasmic material [20]. The chromosomes should not overlap. This can be avoided after optimization the concentration of the cell suspension.

3. Use small slide boxes (10–25 slides). During defrosting the slides, leave the box closed on the bench until room temperature reached.

4. The Carnoy's fixative, methanol–acetic acid, 3:1, should be always cold. Before starting the fixation put the Coplin jar containing the fixative in an ice bucket filled with ice for 10 min to reach the temperature, always make the fixative fresh [19].

5. Optimal amounts of pepsin will always require pilot hybridization but, generally frozen sections 5–10 µl for 1–2 min, and paraffin sections 10–20 µl for 2–4 min. Older slides, and tissues within a large stromal component (e.g., more protein) will require much more pepsin for optimization.

6. Other DNA labeling methods are described in detail by [20]. In our laboratory, we use the modified nick translation.

7. Check the temperature during nick translation because it influences the enzyme reaction, add small amount of ice if the temperature starts to increase.

8. There are other suppliers for CCND1 DNA-specific probes.

Acknowledgments

This publication was supported by the National Research Development and Innovation Fund (grant number K112327) and the GINOP-2.3.2-15-2016-00005 project, the project is cofinanced by the European Regional Development Fund.

References

1. Fu M et al (2004) Minireview: cyclin D1: normal and abnormal functions. Endocrinology 145(12):5439–5447

2. Kim JK, Diehl JA (2009) Nuclear cyclin D1: an oncogenic driver in human cancer. J Cell Physiol 220(2):292–296

3. Ramirez JA et al (2005) Cyclin D1 expression in melanocytic lesions of the skin. Ann Diagn Pathol 9(4):185–188

4. Diehl JA (2002) Cycling to cancer with cyclin D1. Cancer Biol Ther 1(3):226–231

5. Elsheikh S et al (2008) CCND1 amplification and cyclin D1 expression in breast cancer and their relation with proteomic subgroups and patient outcome. Breast Cancer Res Treat 109(2):325–335

6. Vizkeleti L et al (2012) The role of CCND1 alterations during the progression of cutaneous malignant melanoma. Tumour Biol 33(6):2189–2199

7. Gerami P et al (2011) Copy number gains in 11q13 and 8q24 [corrected] are highly linked to prognosis in cutaneous malignant melanoma. J Mol Diagn 13(3):352–358

8. Akervall J et al (2003) The gene ratios c-MYC:cyclin-dependent kinase (CDK)N2A and CCND1:CDKN2A correlate with poor prognosis in squamous cell carcinoma of the head and neck. Clin Cancer Res 9(5):1750–1755

9. Monteiro E et al (2004) Cyclin D1 A870G polymorphism and amplification in laryngeal squamous cell carcinoma: implications of tumor localization and tobacco exposure. Cancer Detect Prev 28(4):237–243

10. Lazar V et al (2009) Characterization of candidate gene copy number alterations in the 11q13 region along with BRAF and NRAS mutations in human melanoma. Mod Pathol 22(10):1367–1378

11. Bockmuhl U et al (2000) Genetic imbalances with impact on survival in head and neck cancer patients. Am J Pathol 157(2):369–375

12. Izzo JG et al (2003) Cyclin D1 genotype, response to biochemoprevention, and progression rate to upper aerodigestive tract cancer. J Natl Cancer Inst 95(3):198–205

13. Ooi A et al (2016) Gene amplification of CCNE1, CCND1 and CDK6 in gastric cancers detected by multiplex ligation-dependent probe amplification and fluorescence in situ hybridization. Hum Pathol 61:58–67

14. Gerami P (2012) A highly specific and discriminatory FISH assay for distinguishing between benign and malignant melanocytic neoplasms. Am J Surg Pathol 36(6):808–817

15. Ponti G et al (2013) Fluorescence in-situ hybridization and dermoscopy in the assessment of controversial melanocytic tumors. Melanoma Res 23(6):474–480

16. Andreeff M, Pinkel D (1999) Introduction to fluorescence in situ hybridization: principles and clinical applications. Wiley-Liss, New York, p xi, 455

17. Saunders K, Czepulkowski B (2001) Culture of human cells for chromosomal analysis in analyzing chromosomes. BIOS Scientific Publishers, Oxford, UK

18. Dogan S et al (2013) Use of touch imprint cytology as a simple method to enrich tumor cells for molecular analysis. Cancer Cytopathol 121(7):354–360

19. Preparation of paraffin sections and frozen tissue for FISH (2006). Available from: https://ccr.cancer.gov/sites/default/files/preparation_of_paraffin_sections_and_frozen_tissue_for_fish.pdf

20. Garimberti E, Tosi S (2010) Fluorescence in situ hybridization (FISH), basic principles and methodology. Methods Mol Biol 659:3–20

21. Deng W et al (2003) A new method for improving metaphase chromosome spreading. Cytometry A 51(1):46–51

Detection of CCND1 Gene Copy Number Variations Using Multiplex Ligation-Dependent Probe Amplification and Fluorescence In Situ Hybridization Methods

Akishi Ooi and Takeru Oyama

Abstract

The *CCND1* locus is located in 11q13 and encodes the G1–S regulatory protein, cyclin D1. Cyclin D1 is frequently amplified in various types of cancers, and is an attractive potential therapeutic target. Multiplex ligation-dependent probe amplification (MLPA) is a new, high-resolution method for the detection of amplification of numerous genes including *CCND1* in small amounts of DNA fragments derived from formalin-fixed, paraffin-embedded material in a single reaction. This approach is, however, based on PCR and averages many different cells, so validation by morphological methods such as fluorescence in situ hybridization (FISH) is theoretically mandatory. Here we describe detection of *CCND1* gene copy number variations by commercially available MLPA kits and FISH using a bacterial artificial chromosome (BAC) probe.

Key words Formalin-fixed, paraffin-embedded material, Commercially available MLPA kits, BAC probe

1 Introduction

Under normal circumstances, growth factor signaling leads to the expression of cyclin D1 and its complexing with cyclin-dependent kinase 4 (CDK4) or CDK6. Following accumulation of active cyclin D1/CDK4 or CyclinD1/CDK6, CDK2 in combination with cyclin E then accumulates to facilitate the transition from G1 to S phase by phosphorylation of downstream targets, including the tumor suppressor RB [1]. *CCND1* is amplified in various types of cancer such as head and neck, endometrium, pancreas, breast, and stomach [2]. Cyclin D1 is generally regarded as difficult to target directly with therapies, as it lacks intrinsic enzymatic activity and is intracellular. Thus, its functionality may most readily be targeted via their partner kinases, CDK4 or CDK6 [3]. In molecularly targeted therapies, establishing feasible screening methods to identify eligible patients is crucial. Compared to SNP, aCGH and

Pedro G. Santiago-Cardona (ed.), *The Retinoblastoma Protein*, Methods in Molecular Biology, vol. 1726, https://doi.org/10.1007/978-1-4939-7565-5_10, © Springer Science+Business Media, LLC 2018

next-generation sequencing techniques, multiplex ligation-dependent probe amplification (MLPA) is a relatively cheap, easy-to-perform method that allows simultaneous detection of multiple gene copy-number aberrations in small amounts of DNA fragments derived from formalin-fixed material [4]. This approach is, however, based on PCR and averages many different cells, so validation by morphological methods such as fluorescence in situ hybridization (FISH) is theoretically mandatory [5].

2   Materials

In the following list of materials and in their associated procedures, we mention a specific supplier for some of the kits and reagents. There may be acceptable products from other suppliers. However, when specific reagents from vendors are mentioned in the methods, this means that we have optimized the procedures for these particular reagents.

2.1   MLPA

1. MLPA kits containing probes enumerating *CCND1* copy number are commercially available from MRC-Holland (Amsterdam, The Netherlands): P175-A2 Tumor-Gain®, P458-B1 Gastric Cancer®, and P078-C1 Breast cancer®.

2. H_2O: distilled water is filtered with Water Purification System of Millipore and autoclaved.

3. 1 M NaSCN: dissolve 8 g sodium thiocyanate in 1 l of H_2O.

4. TE buffer: Mix 1 M Tris–HCl with an appropriate pH and 0.5 M EDTA pH 8.0, and adjust the final concentrations of Tris–HCl to 10 mM and EDTA to 1 mM.

5. 1 M Tris–HCl: dissolve 121.1 g of Tris base in 800 ml of H_2O. Adjust to the desired pH by adding concentrated HCl. Adjust the volume of the solution to 1 l with H_2O.

6. 0.5 M EDTA pH 8.0: Add 186.1 g of disodium EDTA·$2H_2O$ to 800 ml of H_2O. Adjust pH to 8.0 with NaOH.

7. Proteinase K PCR grade.

8. 20× SSC: Dissolve 175.3 g NaCl, 88.2 g tri-sodium citrate dehydrate in 800 ml distilled water, adjust the pH to 7.0 with 1 N HCl, and adjust to 1 l with H_2O.

9. Coplin jars.

10. 100% xylene.

11. 100% ethanol.

2.2   FISH

1. LB medium: Dissolve 10 g Bacto tryptone, 5 g Bacto yeast extract, and 10 g NaCl in 950 ml distilled water, adjust the pH

to 7.0 with 5 N NaOH. Adjust the volume of the solution to 1 l with distilled water. Sterilize by autoclaving.

2. Qiagen plasmid Mini kit®. This includes P1®, P2® and P3 buffer, as well as QIAGEN tip 20®, Buffer QBT®, and Buffer QC®.

3. Kimwipes®.

4. Nick translation kit: Abbott Laboratories (Abbott Park, IL, USA).

5. 1 μg/μl Cot 1 DNA.

6. 1 μg/μl Human placental DNA.

7. 1 μg/μl *E. coli* tRNA.

8. MAS-coated glass slides: Matsunami, (Tokyo, Japan).

9. 100 mg/ml RNase A.

10. ThermoBrite Kit: Abbott Laboratories (Abbott Park, IL, USA).

11. Protease II®.

12. 100% formamide.

13. NP-40 or Igepal® CA-680 detergent.

14. Locus Specific Identifier DNA probe (LSI): Abbott Laboratories (Abbott Park, IL, USA).

15. DAPI-II®Anti fade® solution, Abbott Laboratories (Abbott Park, IL, USA).

16. Chloroform.

17. Filter paper.

18. 70%, 85%, and 100% ethanol.

19. Phosphate Buffered Saline solution (PBS): the standard recipe for 1 l of 1× PBS consists of 8 g NaCl, 0.2 g KCl, 1.44 g Na_2HPO_4, and 0.24 g KH_2PO_4. Dissolve in 800 ml H_2O, adjust pH to 7.4 with HCl, and complete final volume of 1 l with H_2O. Dispense into aliquots and sterilize either by autoclaving (20 min at 15 PSI) or by filtering.

20. Pretreatment Solution® (Abbott Laboratories, Abbott Park, IL, USA).

21. Isopropanol.

22. 0.2 N HCl.

23. 3 M sodium acetate: Dissolve 246.1 g of sodium acetate in 500 ml of deionized H_2O. Adjust the pH to 5.2 with glacial acetic acid. Allow the solution to cool overnight. Adjust the pH once more to 5.2 with glacial acetic acid. Adjust the final volume to 1 l with deionized H_2O and filter-sterilize.

3 Methods

3.1 MLPA

DNA is extracted from formalin-fixed, paraffin-embedded (FFPE) tissue according to the manufacturer's protocol (Extraction Protocol for DNA from FFPE Tissues, MRC-Holland) with some modifications.

1. Cut three to four 6 μm sections and put them on uncoated slides. Several adjacent 4 μm sections on MAS-coated slides are used for HE, FISH and IHC.

2. Trim the examined area referring to the adjacent HE section, remove unnecessary areas with a razor blade.

3. Heat the slides at 75 °C for 15 min on hot plate to melt the paraffin.

4. Deparaffinize in Coplin jar consecutively in 100% xylene two times 5 min each, in 100% ethanol two times for 30 s each, then wash in water.

5. Remove excess water from the glass slide.

6. Drop 50–100 μl 1 M NaSCN on the section and leave for a few minutes.

7. Peel the section from the glass slide by a spatula, and transfer to 1.5 ml Eppendorf's tube with 1 M NaSCN. Incubate at 37 °C, overnight.

8. Centrifuge at 15,000 rpm in a benchtop microcentrifuge for 10 min. Discard supernatant, then add distilled water and leave for a few minutes.

9. Centrifuge at 15,000 rpm in a benchtop microcentrifuge for 10 min. Discard supernatant and add TE buffer pH 7.2. Tap and leave for a few minutes.

10. Centrifuge at 15,000 rpm in a benchtop microcentrifuge for 10 min. Discard supernatant. Add 50–100 μl of 0.5 mg/ml proteinase K and incubate at 55 °C overnight.

11. Inactivate proteinase K by incubation at 80 °C for 20 min.

12. Centrifuge at 1000 rpm in a benchtop microcentrifuge for 10 min. Transfer the supernatant to new tube.

13. Measure OD 280/260 by NanoDrop 2000 or equivalent instrument and adjust DNA concentration to 30–40 ng/μl using TE buffer pH 8.2.

DNA denaturation, hybridization reaction, ligation reaction and PCR reaction are done using the thermocycler program for the MLPA reaction exactly according to the "MLPA DNA Protocol version MDP-005; last revised on 22 SEPT 2014" (MRC-Holland). Reaction products are separated by capillary sequencer ABI-310 (Applied Biosystems, Foster City, CA, USA). The DATA are analyzed by Coffalyser (MRC-Holland).

3.2 FISH

For designing FISH probes, generally gene specific Bacterial Artificial Chromosomes (BAC) probes are searched using UCSC Genome Browser or NCBI map viewer, and the LB agars stabbed with *E. coli* carrying BAC probe are available through BACPAC resources (Oakland, CA, USA). In our previous studies, we used RP11-300I6 (69,226,211–69,387,715) which covers *CCND1* (chromosomal position: 69,228,876–69,242,171). Fluorescein-labeled ready-for-use probes for *CCND1* are also commercially available from Abbott Laboratories (Abbott Park, IL, USA).

3.2.1 Extraction and Purification of BAC DNA

1. Spread bacterial suspension by streaking surface of the agar plate with the appropriate antibiotics.

2. After overnight-culture of the plate at 37 °C, pick up a single colony and transfer it to 3 ml of LB medium with antibiotics in 50 ml tube, and incubate at 37 °C for 8 h in 160 rpm, in a shaking incubator.

3. Transfer 50 µl of the culture medium to 50 ml LB medium with antibiotics in 300 ml flask and incubate at 37 °C overnight at 160 rpm, in a shaking incubator.

4. Transfer the culture medium to 50 ml tubes and centrifuge 2200 × *g* for 10 min at 4 °C.

5. Discard the supernatant. Add 6 µl of RNase dissolved in 6 ml of P1 buffer® and mix by Vortex.

6. Add 6 ml of P2 buffer®. Invert 4–5 times to mix and let stand for 5 min.

7. Add 6 ml of P3 buffer®. Invert 4–5 times to mix and let stand on ice 15 min. Repeat this step a total of three times.

8. Add 130 ml of chloroform and transfer to centrifuge tube. Centrifuge at 24,000 × *g* at 4 °C for 20 min.

9. Filter the solution by filter paper. Add 18 ml of isopropyl alcohol to the supernatant and mix it lightly.

10. Centrifuge at 24,000 × *g* at 4 °C for 40 min to 1 h.

11. Discard the supernatant. Stand the tube in an inverted position on a paper towel to allow all the fluid to drain away. Remove any drops of fluid adhering to the wall of the tube by Kimwipes®. Do not allow the pellet to dry completely.

12. Dissolve the precipitate with 300 µl of TE buffer pH 7.0.

13. Equilibrate a QIAGEN-tip 20® by applying 1 ml Buffer QBT®, and allow column to empty by gravity flow.

14. Apply the supernatant from **step 12** to the QIAGEN-tip® and allow it to enter the resin by gravity flow.

15. Wash the QIAGEN–tip® with 2 ml Buffer QC® two times. Allow Buffer QC® to move through the QIAGEN-tip® by gravity flow.

16. Elute DNA with 0.8 ml Buffer QF® prewarmed to 65 °C onto a clean 2 ml vessel.

17. Precipitate DNA by adding 0.56 ml (0.7 volume) of room-temperature isopropanol to the eluted DNA and mix. Centrifuge at >15,000 rpm in a benchtop microcentrifuge for 30 min at 4 °C. Carefully decant the supernatant.

18. Wash the DNA pellet with 1 ml room-temperature 70% ethanol and centrifuge at >15,000 rpm in a benchtop microcentrifuge for 10 min. Carefully decant supernatant.

19. Air-dry pellet by speed vacuum for 5–8 min (we use the Centrifugal Concentrator® CC-101, Tomy, Tokyo, Japan).

20. Resuspend the pellet in 20 μl of TE buffer pH 8.5.

21. Measure the DNA content and adjust the concentration to 1 μg/μl.

3.2.2 Nick Translation Procedure

1. Place a microcentrifuge tube on ice and allow the tube to cool.

2. Add the following components from the Nick translation Kit® to the tube in the order listed below. Briefly centrifuge and vortex the tube *before* adding the nick translation enzyme (which should be the last component to be added in the mix). This procedure can label up to 1 μg of extracted BAC DNA which is enough for ten FISH experiments (one target area equal to 22 × 22 mm). It is important that you *add these components strictly in the order in which they are listed below*.

   – 16.5 μl of dH$_2$O.

   – 1 μl of 1 μg/μl BAC DNA.

   – 25 μl of 0.2 mM fluorescence-labeled dUTP.

   – 5 μl of 0.1 mM dTTPs.

   – 10 μl of 0.1 mM dNTP mix.

   – 5 μl of 10× nick translation buffer.

   – 10 μl of the Nick translation Enzyme.

   Briefly centrifuge and vortex the tube.

3. Incubate at 15 °C for 5–10 h.

4. Stop the reaction by heating in a 70 °C water bath for 3 min. Chill on ice.

5. Ethanol precipitation: Add these components to the tube and vortex briefly.

Reaction solution of **step 2**	50 μl
1 μg/μl cot 1 DNA	10 μl
1 μg/μl human placental DNA	20 μl
1 μg/μl *E. coli* tRNA	10 μl
dH$_2$O	30 μl

6. Add 12 ml (1/10 v) 3 M Sodium Acetate and 300 ml (2.5 v) of 100% ethanol. Briefly vortex and centrifuge. Keep at −80 °C for 1 h. Centrifuge at 15,000 rpm at 4 °C for 30 min in a benchtop microcentrifuge.

7. Discard the supernatant. Air-dry the pellet by speed vacuum for 5–8 min. Suspend the pellet in 10 μl of H_2O.

8. Keep in freezer in dark.

3.2.3 Dual-Color FISH on Formalin-Fixed and Paraffin-Embedded Specimens

1. Place 4 μm-thick sections onto the MAS-coated glass slides®. Mark hybridization areas with a diamond-tipped scriber on the bottom of the specimen slide.

2. Deparaffinize the section by three successive 10-min washes in 100% xylene, followed by three 5-min washes in absolute ethanol.

3. Air-dry the slides and incubate in 0.2 N HCl at room temperature for 20 min.

4. Wash slides in distilled water for 3 min.

5. Wash slides in 2× SSC for 3 min.

6. Incubate slides in a glass Coplin jar containing 40 ml of the Pretreatment Solution® at 80 °C for 30 min, followed by 1-min wash in distilled water and two 5-min washes in 2× SSC.

7. Incubate slides in RNase A (100 μg/ml in 2× SSC) at 37 °C for 30 min using ThermoBrite®.

8. Wash slides in 2× SSC two times for 5 min each.

9. Prepare a 5 mg/ml protease solution by dissolving 5 mg of Protease II® in 1 ml of 0.01 N HCl. Incubate slides in 100 μl of Protease II solution at 37 °C for 30 min using ThermoBrite®.

10. Wash slides in 2× SSC two times for 5 min each.

11. Rinse slides in 10% buffered formalin in PBS at room temperature for 10 min.

12. Wash slides in 2× SSC two times for 5 min each.

13. Dehydrate the slide in successive rinses in 70%, 85%, 100% ethanol for 2 min each.

14. Allow slides to air-dry.

15. Probe preparation (*see* **Note 1**): Add the following components to the Eppendorf tube. This procedure labels 10 μl of the probe solution, which is enough for a FISH experiment (one target area equal to 22 × 22 mm).

Gene-specific probe	1 μl
CEP 11probe®	1 μl
ddH₂O	1 μl
LSI/WCP hybridization buffer®	7 μl

Total reaction volume is 10 μl. Briefly centrifuge and vortex the tube.

16. Apply probe and seal cover glass by paper bond.

17. For denaturation and hybridization, heat slides at 75 °C for 5 min and incubate slides at 37 °C overnight.

18. Do post hybridization washes by washing slides in 40 ml of 50% formamide/2× SSC in a Coplin jar at 45 °C three times for 10 min each. You can prepare this solution by mixing 20 ml 100% formamide with 20 ml of 4× SSC.

19. Wash slides in 2× SSC, at 45 °C for 10 min.

20. Rinse the slides in 40 ml of 0.1% NP-40/2× SSC, at 45 °C for 10 min. You can prepare this solution by adding 0.4 ml of 10% NP-40 in 39.6 ml of 2× SSC.

21. Rinse slides in 2× SSC at room temperature two times, 5 min each.

22. After air drying, add DAPI-II®/Anti fade® solution, and cover slide with a cover slip. Put slides in suitable boxes, which should be kept at −20 °C before observation.

23. Examine slides with a fluorescence microscope equipped with Triple Bandpass Filter sets® (Abbott) or equivalent for DAPI II, SpectrumOrange®, and SpectrumGreen® (*see* **Note 2**).

4   Notes

1. To detect a numerical aberration of a gene, dual-color FISH is applied: a centromeric probe can be used as a reference probe to assist in distinguishing real gene amplification from an increased gene number resulting from chromosomal polysomy at which the gene is located. Some fluorescence-labeled centromeric specific probes are commercially available.

2. The critical step in FISH using paraffin-embedded tissue is the removal of nuclear protein by enzymatic digestion. The optimal digestion condition may be modified to accommodate each section, because fixation conditions can be different for various individual specimens. If FISH signals look blurred in white cloudy nuclei instead of DAPI-positive blue nuclei, additional digestion may remarkably improve the image. This can be done as follows: remove the coverslip in 2× SSC, followed by heat-denaturing of the probes (this is done by incubating slides in 50% formamide/2× SSC at 75 °C for 15 min in a Coplin jar). Then, wash slides in 2× SSC two times for 5 min each. Go back to the Protease (**step 9**, Subheading 3.2.3) and digest for an additional time of 20–60 min and follow the subsequent steps.

References

1. Etemadmoghadam D, Au-Yeung G, Wall M, Mitchell C, Kansara M, Loehrer E et al (2013) Resistance to CDK2 inhibitors is associated with selection of polyploid cells in CCNE1-amplified ovarian cancer. Clin Cancer Res 19:5960–5971
2. Musgrove EA, Caldon CE, Barraclough J, Stone A, Sutherland RL (2011) Cyclin D as a therapeutic target in cancer. Nat Rev Cancer 11:558–572
3. Ismail A, Bandla S, Reveiller M, Toia L, Zhou Z, Gooding WE et al (2011) Early G(1) cyclin-dependent kinases as prognostic markers and potential therapeutic targets in esophageal adenocarcinoma. Clin Cancer Res 1713:4513–4522
4. Moelans CB, van der Groep P, Hoefnagel LD, van de Vijver MJ, Wesseling P, Wesseling J et al (2014) Genomic evolution from primary breast carcinoma to distant metastasis: few copy number changes of breast cancer related genes. Cancer Lett 344:138–146
5. Ooi A, Oyama T, Nakamura R, Tajiri R, Ikeda H, Fushida S et al (2015) Semi-comprehensive analysis of gene amplification in gastric cancers using multiplex ligation-dependent probe amplification and fluorescence in situ hybridization. Mod Pathol 28:861–871

Chapter 11

Detection of p16 Promoter Hypermethylation by Methylation-Specific PCR

Javed Hussain Choudhury, Raima Das, Shaheen Laskar, Sharbadeb Kundu, Manish Kumar, Partha Pratim Das, Yashmin Choudhury, Rosy Mondal, and Sankar Kumar Ghosh

Abstract

DNA methylation plays a decisive role in the regulation and control of gene expression. DNA methylation is a covalent modification, in which a methyl group is attached to the 5th carbon of the cytosine ring of a CpG dinucleotide that is located upstream from the promoter region of a gene. Promoter hypermethylation (gain of DNA methylation) of the *p16* gene may cause silencing of gene expression and plays an important role in cancer. Therefore, detection of the methylation status of *p16* gene is an important tool in epigenetic studies of various human cancers. The methylation-specific PCR (MSP) is the most commonly used technique for studying DNA methylation. This technique is based on bisulfite modification of DNA, which converts unmethylated cytosine (C) into uracil (U) and leaving methylated cytosine (C^m) unchanged. Here we describe the bisulfite modification of DNA samples and detection of promoter methylation of *p16* gene from bisulfite-treated DNA using MSP. In MSP, modified DNA samples are subjected to PCR amplification using methylated and unmethylated specific primers for the *p16* gene separately. The PCR amplified products are then analyzed in a 2.5–3% agarose gel containing ethidium bromide. The PCR amplified band generated by specific sets of primers is used to determine the methylation status of the *p16* gene.

Key words DNA methylation, *p16* gene hypermethylation, Bisulfite modification, Specific primers, Methylation-specific PCR, Agarose gel electrophoresis

1 Introduction

DNA methylation plays a crucial role in the regulation and control of gene expression. DNA methylation is a covalent modification, in which a methyl group is attached to the 5th carbon of the cytosine ring of a CpG dinucleotide (at CpG Islands) by the enzyme DNA methyltransferases (DNMTs). The CpG dinucleotide is located upstream from the promoter region of a gene [1]. Promoter hypermethylation (gain of DNA methylation) can cause silencing of tumour suppressor's pathway genes (such as *p16*, *p53*, *DAPK*, *ECAD*, and *RASSF1A*) in various human cancers. Therefore,

Pedro G. Santiago-Cardona (ed.), *The Retinoblastoma Protein*, Methods in Molecular Biology, vol. 1726, https://doi.org/10.1007/978-1-4939-7565-5_11, © Springer Science+Business Media, LLC 2018

detection of promoter methylation of tumor suppressing genes has turned out to be an important tool for early diagnostics of cancer [2–5]. Bisulfite modification is the most widely used method for methylation analysis. It is the "gold standard" for DNA methylation study and assists detection and quantification of methylation at single nucleotide resolution. In bisulfite modification or treatment of genomic DNA, unmethylated cytosine (C) converts or modifies into uracil (U), whereas methylated cytosine (C^m) remains unchanged. This bisulfite modification allows us to differentiate methylated DNA from unmethylated DNA [6]. The basic mechanism by which this process is driven starts with the nucleophilic addition of bisulfite to the 6th carbon position of unmethylated cytosine, which allows the swift deamination of cytosine into 5,6-dihydrouracil-6-sulfonate. Following treatment with an alkaline solution quickly removes the sulfonate group and reinforces the double bond thus yielding uracil. However, in the case of methylated cytosines, this reaction is blocked due to the tremendously low reaction rates for the formation of 5-methyl-6-dihydrocytosine-6-sulfonate, and thus they are not converted to uracil. Different techniques have been used based on bisulfite modification for detection of the methylation pattern of genes, such as bisulfite sequencing, combined bisulfite restriction analysis (COBRA), methylation-specific PCR (MSP), real-time MSP or MethyLight, pyrosequencing, and MassArray. All these methods are primarily based on principles that differentially recognize 5-methylcytosine (C^m) from cytosine (C) [7]. During the downstream process, such as methylation specific PCR (MSP) or bisulfite sequencing, unmethylated cytosines are read as thymines and methylated cytosines still read as cytosines (since it is resistant to the bisulfite conversion) (Fig. 1) [8, 9]. In early days, bisulfite modification methods to explore DNA methylation involved an overnight bisulfite treatment step, and in the process, DNA was rigorously damaged. Nowadays commercial kits are available which take only a few hours to complete and often yield less fragmented DNA compared to conventional old methods. These commercially available kits make the bisulfite treatment process very simple and offer >99.5% conversion efficiency of unmethylated cytosines, with almost no conversion of methylated cytosine.

During the bisulfite modification process, DNA is chemically denatured to allow bisulfite reagent to react specifically with single-stranded DNA, as a result deaminating cytosine and creating a uracil residue. DNA denaturation and bisulfite modification is carried out simultaneously. The unique DNA protection reagents in the modification buffer prevent chemical and thermophilic degradation of DNA in the bisulfite treatment. These bisulfite-treated DNA samples are used to perform methylation-specific PCR as well as sequencing, which explore the DNA methylation pattern. The most common method for methylation study is

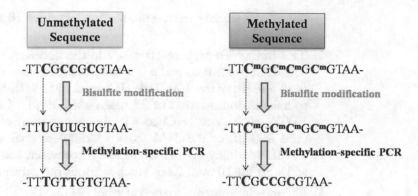

Fig. 1 Bisulfite modification and methylation-specific PCR. In bisulfite modification DNA, cytosine (C) from unmethylated sequence is converted to uracil (U), whereas in methylated cytosine (C^m) remains unchanged. In PCR amplification, uracil (U) is amplified as thymine (T) while methylated cytosine (C^m) remain as cytosine (C), allowing methylated sequence to be distinguished from un-methylated by presence of a cytosine (C) versus thymine (T)

methylation-specific PCR (MSP), which utilizes the cytosine (C) to uracil (U) change and uses primers that will anneal based on those nucleotide changes. In methylation-specific PCR (MSP), two separate sets of primers are designed for detection of methylation. Since the two strands of DNA are no longer complementary after bisulfite treatment, primers can be designed for either modified strand. Therefore, we can use both methylated and unmethylated specific primers for the *p16* gene. The PCR amplified band generated by specific sets of primers will determine the methylation status of the DNA sample. The flexibility of MSP in selecting a genomic segment is very large because PCR primers can be designed at any position [10, 11].

2   Materials

All chemicals used in this procedure should be of molecular grade.

2.1 Stock Solutions and Buffers for DNA Isolation

1. 1 M Tris–HCl, pH 8.0: To prepare 10 mL, add 1.211 g of Trisma base to 7 mL of nuclease-free water, and adjust the pH to 8.00 by adding concentrated HCl. After adjusting the pH, complete the volume to 10 mL with nuclease-free water.

2. 0.5 M EDTA, pH 8.0: To prepare 10 mL, add 1.862 g of EDTA to 7 mL of distilled water, and adjust the pH to 8.0 with NaOH. Complete with water to a final volume of 10 mL, autoclave at 15 psi for 10 min. Keep stock at 22 °C.

3. 5 M NaCl: To prepare 10 mL, add 2.422 g of NaCl to 10 mL of distilled water, and mix until complete dissolution of the

salt using a sterile stirrer. Autoclave at 15 psi for 10 min. Keep stock at 22 °C.

4. TES Buffer: To prepare 10 mL, add the necessary volume of Tris–HCl pH 8.0 to make it a final concentration of 50 mM (add 500 μL of the 1 M Trsi–HCl stock, pH 8.0), add EDTA to a final concentration of 25 mM (add 500 μL of the 0.5 M EDTA stock), and NaCl to a final concentration of 150 mM (add 300 μL of the 5 M stock). Complete final volume to 10 mL by adding 8.7 mL of nuclease-free water, and autoclave at 15 psi for 10 min. Keep stock at room temperature (RT).

5. Phenol–chloroform–isoamyl alcohol (25:24:1).

6. Proteinase K solution 20 mg/mL.

7. 10% SDS solution.

8. Ethanol, 70% and 100%.

2.2 Bisulfite DNA Modification

We use The Imprint® DNA Modification Kit (Sigma-Aldrich, USA; Catalog Number MOD50) for bisulfite modification of DNA samples. The kit contains all the reagents necessary for complete bisulfite conversion and subsequent purification of DNA samples. The contents of this kit should provide for 50 reactions and should be the following:

1. DNA Modification Powder (5 vials).

2. DNA Modification Solution (6.5 mL).

3. Balance Solution (0.5 mL).

4. Ethanol Wash Solution. Prepare by adding 10 μL of Balance Solution to 1.1 mL of 90% ethanol.

5. Capture Solution (20 mL).

6. Cleaning Solution (3.5 mL). Before using this solution, you need to dilute with ethanol by adding 8.2 mL of absolute ethanol to the Cleaning solution bottle and mix.

7. Elution Solution (1.5 mL).

8. Spin Column (50 each).

9. Cap-less Collection Tube (50 each, 2 mL per tube).

10. Collection Tube (50 each, 1.5 mL per tube).

11. In addition to the kit's components listed above, you need standard laboratory heating blocks or water baths. For the procedure, have them preset for incubation at 65 °C, and 99 °C. You also need a vortex apparatus.

12. Standard 1.5 mL microcentrifuge tubes.

13. 90% and 100% ethanol (for preparing Ethanol Wash Solution and Cleaning Solution, respectively).

Table 1
Primers used for detection of *p16* promoter hypermethylation using methylation-specific PCR. MF, methylated forward; MR, methylated reverse; UF, unmethylated forward; UR, unmethylated reverse

Primer name	Primer sequence	Annealing temperature (°C)	Size (bp)
p16-MF	TTA TTA GAG GGT GGG GCG GATCGC (sense)	150	65
p16-MR	GAC CCC GAA CCG CGA CCG TAA (antisense)		
p16-UF	TTA TTA GAG GGT GGG GTG GATTGT (sense)	151	60
p16-UR	CAA CCC CAA ACC ACA ACC ATA A (antisense)		

2.3 Primers Used for Methylation-Specific PCR (MSP)

1. Design primers to distinguish methylated from unmethylated DNA in bisulfate modified DNA. In Table 1, sequences and other information about primers for detection of promoter methylation of *p16* gene are provided.

2.4 Methylation-Sensitive PCR Reaction Mix

1. This reaction mix is prepared by mixing the following components in a total reaction volume of 20 μL: 10 μL of the 2× BioMix™ (Bioline, UK), Forward and Reverse Primers, *add 1 μL of each primer* from stock solutions of 20 pmole/μL, bisulfite modified DNA (use 100–200 ng per reaction mix), and complete to 20 μL with nuclease-free water.

2. Gradient Thermal Cycler.

3. Agarose (for electrophoretic verification of PCR products).

4. Ethidium Bromide solution (for agarose gel staining).

3   Methods

3.1 Genomic DNA Isolation

DNA was isolated from tissue samples using the standard phenol/chloroform procedure as described below.

1. Tissue samples are removed from alcohol and chopped with a sterile blade to small pieces (as small as possible) and then kept dry in −80 °C for 30 min. The samples are then added to a precooled (dry ice) mortar, homogenized gently in 2 volumes (W/V) cold TES buffer. Keep always the homogenate in ice. Adjust the final volume of the homogenate to 500 μL with TES buffer (*see* **Note 1**).

2. Add 50 µL of 10% SDS to the homogenate, followed by adding 5–10 µL of the 20 mg/mL proteinase K stock, and incubate at 56 °C for 1–18 h until the tissue is totally dissolved (*see* **Note 2**).

3. Add an equal volume of phenol–chloroform–isoamyl alcohol (25:24:1), and mix thoroughly for a few minutes.

4. Centrifuge for 10 min at 12,000 rpms in a benchtop microcentrifuge.

5. Transfer the upper phase to a clean 1.5 mL tube and add an equal volume of chloroform–isoamyl alcohol (24:1), and centrifuge again for 10 min at 12,000 rpms in a benchtop microcentrifuge (*see* **Note 3**).

6. Transfer upper aqueous phase to a clean sterile tube and add two volumes of chilled absolute ethanol.

7. Allow the DNA to precipitate overnight at −20 °C.

8. Centrifuge for 10 min at 10,000 rpms in a benchtop microcentrifuge.

9. Carefully remove and discard the supernatant and keep the pellet.

10. Wash the pellet by adding 500 µL of 70% ethanol, followed by centrifugation at 7000 rpms for 10 min. Decant the supernatant.

11. Allow the pellet to air-dry, inside a laminar flow hood.

12. Resuspend the pellet in nuclease-free water and store at −20 °C for further use, or at −80 °C for long-term preservation.

3.2 Determination of the Purity and Yield of the Extracted DNA

1. The DNA isolated to be used for MSP should be pure, i.e., free from most of the associated proteins that keeps DNA coiled and should be in adequate quantity. Therefore, before undergoing downstream process with the extracted DNA, the purity and yield of the DNA must be checked by spectrophotometric and agarose gel electrophoresis procedures (*see* **Notes 4 and 5**).

3.3 Bisulfite Treatment of Genomic DNA (One-Step Modification Procedure)

1. Add 1.1 mL of DNA Modification Solution to 1 vial of DNA Modification Powder. Vortex the vial for 2 min or until the solution is clear. The vial should be examined for any particles that may not be dissolved. If particles can still be seen in the solution, incubate the vial at 65 °C for 2 min and vortex briefly.

2. Add 40 µL of Balance Solution to the vial and vortex briefly.

3. Add 10 µL of DNA to a 1.5 mL micro-centrifuge tube. To this tube, add 110 µL of the solution from **step 1**. Vortex briefly, and then incubate at 99 °C for 6 min.

4. After the incubation, immediately follow with another incubation at 65 °C for 90 min and then proceed to the postmodification DNA cleanup in the next section (*see* **Notes 6** and **7**).

3.4 Postmodification
Cleanup

1. Place a spin column into a 2 mL cap-less collection tube for each sample that was modified.

2. Add 300 µL of Capture Solution to the spin column and allow the solution to sit on the column for 1 min.

3. Add the modified DNA solution from the previous section (Subheading 3.3, Bisulfate Treatment of Genomic DNA) on to the spin column already containing the Capture Solution. Then centrifuge the column at 12,000 × *g* for 20 s. Discard the flow through.

4. Add 200 µL of ethanol-diluted Cleaning Solution to the spin column and centrifuge at 12,000 × *g* for 20 s.

5. Add 50 µL of the Ethanol Wash Solution to the bottom of the spin column. Ensure that air bubbles are not impeding liquid flow to the column filter, and incubate for 8 min at room temperature. After incubation, centrifuge for 20 s and discard the flow through.

6. Add 200 µL of 90% ethanol Solution to the spin column and centrifuge for 20 s and discard the flow through.

7. Again, add 200 µL of 90% ethanol Solution to the Spin Column and centrifuge for 40 s. Discard the 2 mL Cap-less Collection Tube and place the Spin Column into the 1.5 mL Collection Tube.

8. Add 8–20 µL of Elution Solution to the bottom of the Spin Column. Incubate the solution for 1 min and then centrifuge for 20 s. Remove and discard the Spin Column. The eluted solution is the cleaned modified DNA. The modified DNA is now ready for downstream testing or it may be stored at −20 °C for up to 2 months (*see* **Notes 8–14**).

3.5 PCR
Amplification of the
Modified Genomic
DNA by Methylation-
Specific PCR (MSP)

After bisulfite treatment, the modified and cleaned DNA is subjected to PCR amplification using both methylated and unmethylated specific sets of primers. During PCR, unmethylated cytosines amplify as thymines and whereas methylated cytosines amplify as cytosines (Fig. 1). For detection of *p16* promoter hypermethylation by MSP, two primer sets are used (Table 1), the first set of primers recognizes and anneals to methylated sequences of *p16* gene, whereas the second set amplifies unmethylated sequences (alleles). In MSP, the unmethylated and methylated reactions of are carried out separately in reaction mixtures of a total volume of 10 µL each, described below.

1. Set up the PCR reaction indicated in Subheading 2.4. The 2× BioMix™ buffer already contains the Taq DNA polymerase, and thus the reaction only requires the addition of the template, primers and water, as described in Subheading 2.4.

2. Set up positive and negative control reactions. Mix the components of the control reactions exactly as shown in **step 1** of this section for the experimental samples, except for the input DNA, which will vary depending on the control of your choice. As negative control for the unmethylated reaction, we use DNA isolated from peripheral blood of healthy individuals. In the positive control mix for the methylated reaction, we use DNA from peripheral blood treated with *SssI* methyltransferase. You need to use distilled water without template DNA as a negative control in both methylated and unmethylated reactions.

3. Perform all the PCR reactions in a gradient thermal cycler using the following parameters:

Initial denaturation	94 °C for 5 min
Denaturation	94 °C for 1 min
Annealing	Variable (°C) for 45 s
Extension	72 °C for 45 s
Final extension	72 °C for 10 min
Hold	4 °C

3.6 Analysis of MSP Product

1. Analyze the PCR amplified products in 2.5–3% agarose gel containing 10 mg/mL ethidium bromide, running the products of the methylated and unmethylated reactions side-by-side. If the band of expected size is seen on agarose gel electrophoresis, the sample is considered to contain the methylated or unmethylated allele of the gene, depending on the sets of primers used. If a PCR amplified product is generated by primers designed for the methylated site, then we can say the target site is methylated. The band intensity of PCR amplified products generated by the specific primer pairs may vary among samples investigated (Fig. 2). The results from the MSP analysis are visually scored according to three categories such as strongly methylated, moderately methylated and unmethylated. If the analyzed PCR product of DNA samples is of equal or stronger band intensity than the positive control, then the samples are strongly methylated. The bands of PCR products with less intensity than the positive control are classified as moderately methylated, whereas samples with no visible band are considered as unmethylated (*see* **Notes 15–20**).

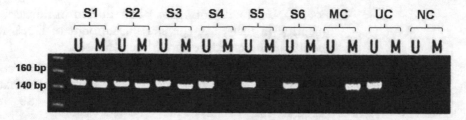

Fig. 2 Ethidium bromide-stained agarose gel electrophoresis for detection of *p16* hypermethylation. PCR-amplified products are designated as unmethylated (**U**), methylated (**M**). Hypermethylated *p16* promoter (**S1**, **S2**, and **S3**); unmethylated *p16* promoter (**S4**, **S5**, and **S6**); **MC** denotes positive control for methylated reaction; **UC** represents positive control for unmethylated reaction and **NC** indicates negative controls

4 Notes

1. During genomic DNA isolation from tissue samples, chopping of tissues into small pieces should be done using sterile techniques. This process can be performed inside a microcentrifuge tube to avoid losing tissue. When using such small tissue samples, static may frequently cause trouble. To avoid static, add 10–20 µL of TES buffer to the sample before chopping.

2. Some tissue samples are hard to digest, in this case repeat the digestion step. It is crucial that tissues are totally digested to ensure maximum yield of DNA.

3. During DNA isolation, special care should be taken to avoid contamination and incomplete phase separation. Make sure that the used chloroform does not contain additives. In case of incomplete phase separation, shake the microcentrifuge tube vigorously for at least 30 s, and repeat the centrifugation step. Bioline Isolate Genomic DNA Minikit (Bioline, UK) or any other appropriate genomic DNA isolation kits could be used as an alternative to the phenol/chloroform extraction procedure.

4. The isolated genomic DNA needs to be of good quality and purity, otherwise, it can hinder the DNA modification process. If the quality and purity of DNA is not good then there is a possibility of DNA damage and breakdown during postmodification cleanup process. Moreover, it may lead to false positive results and misinterpretation of the data. Therefore, quality and purity of genomic DNA should be assessed before bisulfite treatment.

5. For optimal DNA modification procedures, the concentration of the isolated DNA should be in the range of 50–200 ng. For the quality and purity, make sure the DNA A260/280 ratio is between 1.6 and 1.9. The DNA can be checked for degradation by gel electrophoresis. After that, start the downstream analysis only with high quality DNA.

6. Poor DNA modification can occur due to insufficient DNA quantity; in that case, the starting amount of DNA for the modification procedure should be increased.

7. DNA can be poorly modified if the DNA template contains secondary structure or a high G/C contents. In that case, increasing bisulfite treatment time to 150–180 min is recommended.

8. With our procedure, 90 min is sufficient for more than 99% C → U conversion while DNA degradation is greatly prevented. We have observed that increased modification time does not significantly increase C → U conversion, while the yield of modified DNA is significantly reduced most likely due to increased DNA degradation.

9. It is essential to note that in some samples (such as FFPE samples) and samples that underwent fixation protocols, DNA degradation occurs rigorously. For that reason, we recommend amplifying the gene of interest before bisulfite treatment to ensure the integrity of the samples. In this case, it is also recommended use DNA stabilizing reagents, which minimize DNA sample degradation.

10. For best results, the eluted modified DNA should be used without delay, or stored at −20 °C for up to 2 months.

11. During the DNA modification step, always cap the Spin Columns before placing them in a microcentrifuge.

12. All centrifugations during the DNA postmodification cleanup are set at $12,000 \times g$.

13. The Two-Step modification protocol is recommended for low DNA input (100 pg–10 ng). A BSA solution (20 mg/mL) diluted to 0.5 mg/mL (12.5 μL BSA to 487.5 μL of water) can be used as a carrier. The BSA solution will improve DNA recovery when using low input amounts.

14. In the Two-Step Modification procedure, first add DNA sample to a 1.5 mL microcentrifuge tube and adjust the total volume up to 24 μL with prepared 0.5 mg/mL BSA–water solution. Then add 1 μL of Balance Solution. Vortex and incubate the sample at 37 °C for 10 min. Now add 1.1 mL of DNA Modification Solution to 1 vial of DNA Modification Powder, Vortex the vial for 2 min or until the solution is clear. If any particles remain, incubate the vial at 65 °C for 2 min then vortex briefly. Add 40 μL of Balance Solution and vortex briefly. Finally add 125 μL of the prepared solution from **step 2** into the DNA sample after **step 1** incubation. Vortex and incubate at 65 °C for 90 min.

15. Methylation-specific PCR (MSP) is sensitive and specific for methylation of any sites of CpG in a CpG island. The frequency

of CG sites in CpG islands renders this technique uniquely useful and extremely sensitive for such regions. The disadvantage of the technique is the rate of false negative or positive results and thus requires careful determination of the number of PCR cycles to be performed.

16. Effective primer designing for MSP is crucial for specificity and unbiased PCR amplification of modified DNA. Primer should be ~30 bp in length and the annealing temperature above 50 °C. The final base of primers at the 3' end should be a C → T to ensure the amplification of modified DNA.

17. The CpG sites themselves should be avoided in the primer sequences to evade possible bias toward methylated, unmethylated or unconverted DNA templates.

18. PCR amplicons length should be no more than 450 bp to maximize the yield.

19. In the condition where there is a mixture of unmethylated and methylated DNA for a gene of interest, the PCR parameters should be optimized.

20. To optimize PCR parameters, we recommend testing varying annealing temperature, Mg^{2+} concentration, extension time, and primer concentration.

Acknowledgment

The authors are thankful to Cachar Cancer Hospital and Research Centre (CCHRC) and Silchar Medical College and Hospital (SMC), Assam, for providing blood/tissue samples. We are also grateful to the Department of Biotechnology (DBT), Government of India for providing infrastructural facilities.

References

1. Ng HH, Bird A (1999) DNA methylation and chromatin modification. Curr Opin Genet Dev 9(2):158–163

2. Baylin SB (2005) DNA methylation and gene silencing in cancer. Nat Clin Pract Oncol 2(Suppl 1):S4–11. https://doi.org/10.1038/ncponc0354

3. Asokan GS, Jeelani S, Gnanasundaram N (2014) Promoter hypermethylation profile of tumour suppressor genes in oral leukoplakia and oral squamous cell carcinoma. J Clin Diagn Res 8(10):ZC09–ZC12. https://doi.org/10.7860/JCDR/2014/9251.4949

4. Choudhury J, Ghosh S (2015) Promoter hypermethylation profiling identifies subtypes of head and neck cancer with distinct viral, environmental, genetic and survival characteristics. PLoS One 10(6):e0129808

5. Toyota M, Ahuja N, Ohe-Toyota M, Herman JG, Baylin SB, Issa JP (1999) CpG island methylator phenotype in colorectal cancer. Proc Natl Acad Sci U S A 96(15):8681–8686

6. Fraga MF, Esteller M (2002) DNA methylation: a profile of methods and applications. BioTechniques 33(3):632. 634, 636–649

7. Kristensen LS, Hansen LL (2009) PCR-based methods for detecting single-locus DNA methylation biomarkers in cancer diagnostics, prognostics, and response to treatment. Clin Chem 55(8):1471–1483

8. Hayatsu H, Wataya Y, Kazushige K (1970) The addition of sodium bisulfite to uracil and to cytosine. J Am Chem Soc 92(3):724–726

9. Hayatsu H (2008) Discovery of bisulfite-mediated cytosine conversion to uracil, the key reaction for DNA methylation analysis—a personal account. Proc Jpn Acad Ser B Phys Biol Sci 84(8):321–330

10. Herman JG, Graff JR, Myohanen S, Nelkin BD, Baylin SB (1996) Methylation-specific PCR: a novel PCR assay for methylation status of CpG islands. Proc Natl Acad Sci U S A 93(18):9821–9826

11. Shen L, Waterland RA (2007) Methods of DNA methylation analysis. Curr Opin Clin Nutr Metab Care 10(5):576–581

Chapter 12

Immunohistochemical Detection of p16 in Clinical Samples

Georgia Karpathiou and Michel Peoc'h

Abstract

P16 immunohistochemical expression, a surrogate marker of the retinoblastoma pathway, has become a major adjunct in the routine practice mostly of cervical and head/neck pathology, but with other indications too. In this chapter, a detailed immunohistochemical technique for the detection of p16 is described, followed by indications and interpretation of its expression in uterine, ovarian, vulvar, penile, head-and-neck, melanocytic, and other pathologies.

Key words Cervix, Dysplasia, Technique, Immunohistochemistry, Uterus, Melanoma, Interpretation

1 Introduction

Immunohistochemistry (IHC) is the detection of antigens, most often proteins, in tissue sections using antibodies that specifically recognize these antigens. It is thus a protein detection method that offers the unique advantage of detecting the location of these epitopes on tissues and cells. It can be used during routine pathology practice or for research purposes as it is a technique that can be easily adapted in most laboratories without the need of expensive equipment [1–8]. Nowadays, most Pathology Departments are familiar with immunohistochemistry, often as an automated technique, and mostly for diagnostic purposes. One of the most used antibodies during daily practice is the anti-p16 antibody. Its role is central in the management of HPV-associated lesions, but its use is extended to other tumors, too.

During human papilloma virus (HPV) oncogenesis, the retinoblastoma protein (pRB) pathway is altered; normally, when pRB is phosphorylated, it releases the nuclear factor E2F, which then induces the transcription of several genes involved in DNA synthesis (G1 to S switch of the cell cycle) [9]. This event is negatively controlled by p16 and p21. If pRB function is lost, E2F activates constantly its target genes, resulting in nonprogrammed cellular division [9]. The E7 protein produced during HPV infection binds

Pedro G. Santiago-Cardona (ed.), *The Retinoblastoma Protein*, Methods in Molecular Biology, vol. 1726,
https://doi.org/10.1007/978-1-4939-7565-5_12, © Springer Science+Business Media, LLC 2018

and degrades pRB allowing the progression to the S phase. Although p16 levels rise, normal feedback is bypassed [9]. This p16 overexpression is detected immunohistochemically and it can thus be used as an adjunct in diagnosis of HPV-related lesions.

Furthermore, p16 has been found to be overexpressed in various tumor types, in this case showing no association with HPV oncogenesis. P16 is up regulated in the G1 phase of each cell cycle and has an exceptionally long half-life time [10]. In slowly proliferating cells with a doubling time greater than the p16 dismantling period, p16 can be completely cleared from the cell between two mitoses, and thus, p16 staining will be found in only a low fraction of normal proliferating cells [10]. In contrast, rapidly proliferating cancers will show p16 accumulation [10]. In other tumors is the p16 locus, *CDKN2A*, that is disabled. In these cases, like in melanomas or mesotheliomas, is the absence of expression or the detection of the genetic abnormality that provides diagnostic information.

A standard immunohistochemical technique can be used to detect p16 expression in clinical samples. In this case, formalin-fixed, paraffin-embedded tissue (FFPE) is usually used, but frozen sections can be used as well. An automated system is adapted in many Pathology Departments as for most antibodies of the routine practice, but the principles of the technique remain the same, and it can be performed manually. Regarding the monoclonal antibodies used for p16 detection, several clones are used in the literature with E6H4 being often cited. The principles noted below can be used with this clone. Different clones may require different incubation times or epitope retrieval, so assays should be always performed to optimize the conditions [11].

In this chapter, a description of p16 immunohistochemical detection in clinical samples is provided followed by a discussion of the indications of p16 use in clinical pathology.

2   Materials

1. Formalin-fixed, paraffin-embedded tissue. Formalin (water solution of about 40% w/v formaldehyde) is the preferred fixative agent in most Pathology Departments. It is produced by one part of formalin and nine parts of water or buffer producing a 10% formalin solution which contains about 4% formaldehyde w/v, buffered to neutral pH (about 6.8–7.2). This fixative penetrates 1 mm of tissue thickness in an hour. A specimen should not be more than 4 mm thick to optimize fixation and as such larger specimens require sectioning before fixation. Do not forget fixating in an excess of volume of fixative, at least 20:1 fixative to tissue. Embedding of tissue is done in paraffin wax.

2. Microtome and glass slides to perform tissue sectioning after embedding.

3. Ethanol 70% and 95%, these are required for a graded series (baths) of ethanol to be used for dehydration and rehydration of the tissues.

4. Xylene (xylene baths are used for paraffin removal).

5. Antigen or epitope retrieval (ER) can be achieved with two main solutions:

    (a) Citrate buffer (10 mM sodium citrate, 0.05% Tween 20, pH 6.0): 1 L of distilled water, 2.94 g of tri-sodium citrate, add 1 N HCl for adjusting pH to 6.0, and 0.5 mL Tween 20, or

    (b) Tris/EDTA (10 mM Tris base, 1 mM EDTA, 0.05% Tween 20, pH 9.0): 1 L distilled water, 1.21 g Tris base, 0.37 g EDTA, and 0.5 mL Tween 20, adjust pH to 9.0 with HCl.

6. Blocking reagent: 3% H_2O_2

7. Washing buffer, this is Tris buffer normal saline, or TBS: 0.5 M Tris base, 9% (W/V) NaCl, 0.5% Tween 20, pH 8.4. To prepare, mix in 1 L of distilled water 61 g of Trizma base, 90 of NaCl, and 5 mL of Tween 20, adjust pH to 8.4 with HCl. Dilute 1:10 with distilled water before use, and adjust pH after dilution if necessary.

8. Primary antibody.

9. Polymer reagent conjugated with horseradish peroxidase and anti-Fab antibody.

10. DAB (3,3′-diaminobenzidine).

11. Hematoxylin.

12. Drying oven, pressure cooker, appropriate containers, slides racks, baths, distilled/deionized water.

3   Methods

3.1 Immuno-histochemical Staining of p16 in Tissue Samples

1. 3–5 μm thick sections are prepared with the microtome and mounted on positively charged glass slides. These prevent sections from falling off the slide.

2. Place slides in a drying oven at a temperature of 60 °C for 20 min. Water is removed and the section adheres better; also, paraffin melts in this step.

3. The unstained slides must now be deparaffinized and rehydrated. Paraffin must be promptly removed, as residual paraffin will give nonspecific staining. Xylene baths (2 × 5 min) are followed by ethanol baths (2 × 3 min in 95% ethanol and 2 × 3 min

in 70% ethanol). Finish with distilled/deionized water for 30 s (*see* **Note 1**).

4. Fixation masks antigenic sites, so antigen retrieval allows to antigenic sites to be exposed to antibodies. Epitope retrieval (ER) will be heat-induced in the citrate buffer pH 6.0 for 50 min. A pressure cooker can be used for this step. Begin with 95–100 °C for 30 min and allow to cool in room temperature for 20 min, followed by a 5 min in TBS buffer bath (*see* **Notes 2 and 3**). Alternatively, the EDTA-based ER buffer (pH 9.0) can be also used, usually for shorter time (10 min in 100 °C, 20 min to cool). Always perform assays to optimize conditions in your laboratory and under your habits.

5. Apply the 3% hydrogen peroxide (peroxidase blocking reagent) for 5–10 min in room temperature followed by a TBS buffer bath for 5 min. This step blocks endogenous tissue peroxidase, which after inactivation will not compete with the peroxidase that is conjugated to the secondary antibody. This will minimize nonspecific background due to endogenous peroxidase activity.

6. The slides are now ready to be incubated with the primary antibody; cover the slide with 200 μL of the primary antibody for 30 min at room temperature. E6H4 is a monoclonal mouse antibody; commercial kits often contain a ready-to-use prediluted product. If not, a dilution of 1:50–1:100 is usually used. Always follow manufacturer's instructions and perform essays to achieve the best staining. Follow by 5 min TBS buffer bath (*see* **Note 4**).

7. E6H4 clone is a mouse anti-human antibody. This means the secondary antibody must be anti-mouse. Commercial kits are available containing polymer reagent conjugated with horseradish peroxidase and anti-Fab antibody. Cover slides for 30 min with 200 μL of the reagent. Follow with 5 min TBS buffer bath × 2 times (*see* **Note 5**).

8. Use 200 μL of DAB (2,2′ diaminobenzidine, the chromogen that will be converted to a visible brown product after peroxidase action) to cover the slide for 10 min. Rinse with distilled/deionized water (DAB is a hazardous material, so its waste should be properly disposed of in an appropriate container).

9. Counterstain with hematoxylin for 5 min in a hematoxylin bath. Rinse well with tap water and then in distilled/deionized water.

10. Dehydrate (2 × 3 min 70% ethanol, 2 × 3 min 95% ethanol, 2 × 5 min xylene) and mount slides.

3.2   Indications

The following are some indications and interpretations of p16 expression in uterine, ovarian, vulvar, penile, head-and-neck, melanocytic, and other pathologies (*see* **Notes 6** and **7** regarding staining).

3.2.1   Uterine Cervix

P16 immunohistochemistry is widely used in the routine practice of cervical pathology, especially when diagnosing dysplastic lesions. In 2012, the College of American Pathologists and the American Society for Colposcopy and Cervical Pathology published the Lower Anogenital Squamous Terminology or "LAST" recommendations for histopathology reporting of Human Papilloma Virus (HPV)-related squamous lesions of the lower anogenital tract: they recommend the use of a two-tier nomenclature [low-grade squamous intraepithelial lesion (LSIL) and high-grade squamous intraepithelial lesion (HSIL), also adopted by the World Health Organization [12]] and the use of p16 immunohistochemistry to classify equivocal lesions [13]. P16 staining implementation in the routine practice and high grade lesion diagnosis has increased dramatically after LAST recommendations [14]. These recommendations mostly aid in intraepithelial neoplasia (IN)-2 classification as either LSIL or HSIL, as approximately one-third of equivocal IN-2 diagnoses will be downgraded to LSIL, whereas there is a significant association of p16 expression with a higher risk for HSIL on a subsequent specimen [15]. A still open question is whether p16 expression in low grade lesions is actually a prognostic marker of progression, as studies until now give contrasting results [16]. Moreover, p16 staining helps to distinguish HSIL form mimics like atrophy, immature squamous metaplasia, and reparative changes [13].

Thus, when encountering a p16 positive dysplastic cervical lesion, a high grade intraepithelial lesion is generally diagnosed. However, this should be done with caution and with knowledge of the several pitfalls. To begin with, what is considered as positive? The LAST classification defines as positive a continuous strong "block" positivity of nuclei and cytoplasm in at least one third of the epithelium beginning form the base upward. In practice, most really high-grade lesions classified as cervical intraepithelial neoplasia (CIN)-3 will be strongly positive in the whole thickness of the epithelium (Fig. 1a, b). In contrast, the patchy weak staining of some epithelial cells is considered negative (Fig. 1c, d); this kind of staining is often seen with a low-grade lesion either CIN1 or just condylomatous modifications (cases with viral infestation signs like koilocytes, binuclear or multinuclear epithelial cells, koilocytic atypia). In more detail, "block" pattern is defined as strong, continuous, nuclear ± cytoplasmic staining involving at least one-third thickness of the epithelium over a significant distance [17]. Patchy staining is defined as alternating clusters of positively (weak or strong) or negatively stained cells, with positive cells tending to

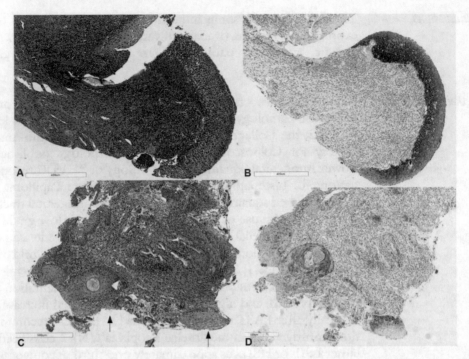

Fig. 1 P16 in squamous intraepithelial lesions. (**a**) A HSIL (CIN3) of the uterine cervix (HES ×60). (**b**) Strong "block" positivity for p16 (×60). (**c**) Squamous cell metaplasia with viral infection signs (arrows) at the squamocolumnar junction with no dysplasia (HES ×50). (**d**) P16 heterogeneous "patchy" mild expression should be interpreted as negative (×50). *HES* hematoxylin, eosin, safranin. All routine slides presented here are HES-stained. All immunohistochemistry slides are counterstained with hematoxylin

reside in the middle or superficial cell layers [17]. A minute pattern of expression can be also seen: strong positive p16 staining but limited to a very small focus or small detached epithelia—<10 cells in length and <5 cell layers in thickness [17].

As mentioned earlier, p16 IHC is mainly used to better classify IN-2 cases (Fig. 2). However, 11.5% of morphologically IN-2 cases—where p16 IHC is mostly used—have discrepant p16 interpretations: (1) diffuse strong staining involving less than the lower third of the epithelium; (2) diffuse staining in at least the lower third of the epithelium but with a weak intensity; (3) a focal area of diffuse staining, which could be interpreted either as a focus of true positivity or as part of a larger pattern of patchy (nondiffuse) staining; and (4) strong extensive staining with intervening negative areas imparting an overall patchy or mosaic pattern [15]. In these cases, correlation with morphology is what will finally guide the correct diagnosis.

Inversely, but similarly representing the pitfalls of p16 overuse, are cases with an initial HSIL diagnosis but a negative follow-up; almost half of them are actually LSIL or nondysplastic lesions misdiagnosed in the basis of p16 IHC either because p16 IHC is overused on unequivocal CIN1 lesions which are then upgraded as

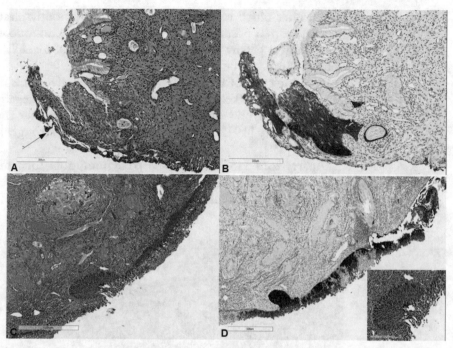

Fig. 2 P16 in squamous intraepithelial lesions. (**a, b**) Dysplastic lesions often arise in metaplastic epithelium (arrow), so attributing a grade is sometimes difficult in regard to the epithelium thickness (HES ×100). P16 strong "block" expression verifies that this is a high-grade lesion (×100). (**c, d**) P16 expression in this cone biopsy is strong but with heterogeneous distribution (×50). Correlation with morphology is imperative to verify that strongly positive foci correspond to high grade lesions (**c**, HES ×50; Inset, HES ×200). *HES* hematoxylin, eosin, safranin. All routine slides presented here are HES-stained. All immunohistochemistry slides are counterstained with hematoxylin

they may show strong, basal/parabasal positive p16 staining or the diagnoses are based on non-block p16 staining patterns, as those previously mentioned [17]. This highlights the problems regarding CIN1 lesions: some of these cases can be strongly positive in the lower third of the epithelium, but they still are low grade lesions. If the biopsy consists of small detached fragments or if the fragments are not well oriented when embedded, then this positivity cannot be judged in relation to the layers of the epithelium, i.e., the correlation with morphology cannot be done. Thus, when finding a squamous intraepithelial lesion in small fragments, tangential cuts, and free-floating single cells it is not always possible to grade it; in these cases, p16 has a sensitivity of 81.6%, a specificity of 35%, a positive predictive value of 54.4%, and a negative predictive value of 66.7% [18].

In all of these cases, confrontation with the morphology is imperative. Having said that, it is suggested to perform p16 immunohistochemistry only when a high grade is suspected by morphology but it is not certain—mostly CIN2 lesions or CIN3 mimics like atrophy—and not in unequivocal CIN1 or CIN3 cases.

Another pitfall regarding p16 IHC is the nondysplastic cells that can be p16 positive; these include endocervical mucosal cells which show a patchy positivity and some cases of metaplastic epithelium which can be also slightly positive.

In some cases of HSIL, HPV testing is negative. This negative HPV status most likely represents the analytical false-negative testing linked to hybrid captured detection method rather than true HPV negativity [19]. In these cases, p16 remains strongly positive for HSIL [19].

Apart from HSIL diagnosis, p16 immunohistochemistry is also used to better assess the margins of a cone biopsy when these are electrocoagulated as expression is retained (Fig. 3).

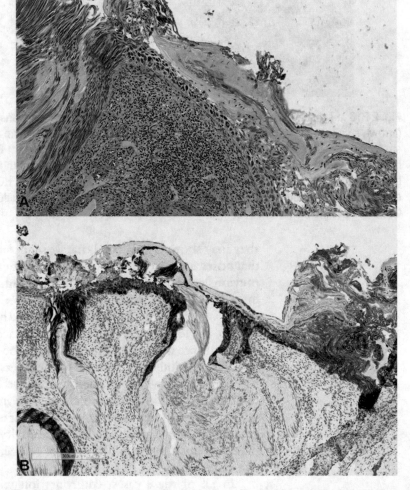

Fig. 3 P16 in squamous intraepithelial lesions. An electrocoagulated cone biopsy margin can be assessed by p16, as high grade lesions retain its expression (**a**, HES ×100; **b**, ×100). HES, hematoxylin, eosin, safranin. All routine slides presented here are HES-stained. All immunohistochemistry slides are counterstained with hematoxylin

P16 immunohistochemistry is also used in the diagnosis of invasive lesions (Fig. 4). The vast majority of cervical squamous cell carcinomas, adenocarcinomas, adenosquamous carcinomas, and neuroendocrine carcinomas express p16. Gastric-type endocervical adenocarcinomas are an exception as they do not harbor HPV DNA neither p16 expression, representing an HPV-independent tumor [20]. In endocervical glandular lesions, p16 is used to exclude an endometrial primary, as this is typically (grade 1 or 2 endometrioid adenocarcinomas) negative for p16. Caution should be exercised as high grade (grade 3) endometrial endometrioid adenocarcinomas as well as serous and clear cell carcinomas

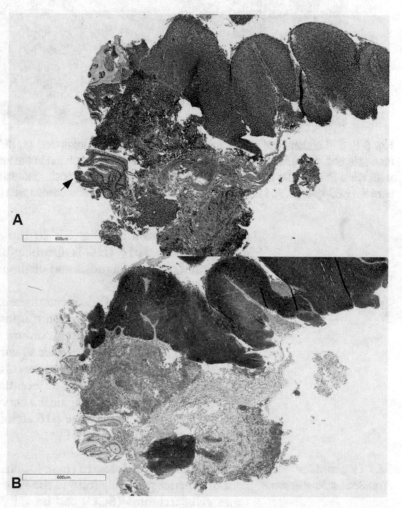

Fig. 4 P16 in anal squamous cell carcinomas. Carcinoma is strongly and diffusely positive for p16 (**a**, HES ×40; **b**, ×40). Normal colonic mucosa (arrow) is negative for p16 (×40). *HES* hematoxylin, eosin, safranin. All routine slides presented here are HES-stained. All immunohistochemistry slides are counterstained with hematoxylin

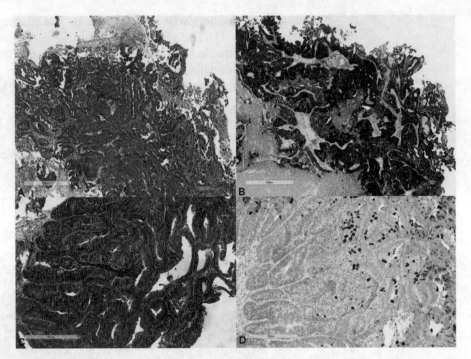

Fig. 5 P16 in endometrial carcinomas. Endometrial serous carcinomas (**a**, HES ×50) may morphologically resemble endometrioid carcinomas (**c**, HES ×100), but p16 expression in the former is strong and diffuse (**b**, ×50) while in the latter is "patchy" (**d**, ×100). HES, hematoxylin, eosin, safranin. All routine slides presented here are HES-stained. All immunohistochemistry slides are counterstained with hematoxylin

are often p16 positive (Fig. 5). In the context of endocervical glandular lesions, p16 IHC is also helpful in establishing an adenocarcinoma in situ diagnosis and distinguishing it from a reactive atypia (Fig. 6).

In some rare cases of advanced disease, the question of a cervical primary can be posed in genitourinary specimens. In these cases, p16 overexpression cannot confirm a cervical primary as it is also found in almost 30% of bladder squamous cell carcinomas and urothelial carcinomas with squamous differentiation [21]. The main utility of p16 IHC in this differential diagnosis is that negative and patchy results argue against a cervical primary, although in a minority of cases, nondiffuse p16 staining does not definitively rule out cervical carcinoma [21].

3.2.2 Vagina/Vulva/ Penis/Scrotum/Anal Region

Despite data are much less in these localizations than in the cervix, routine practice generally follows the same rules [16]. Vulvar squamous cell carcinoma (SCC) can be HPV-associated, which presents in younger women, is associated with the usual type vulvar intraepithelial neoplasia (VIN) and overexpresses p16, or HPV-independent SCCs presenting in older women and being associated with differentiated VIN and lichen sclerosus [22, 23]. P16 expression by vulvar SCCs is associated with a better prognosis [22].

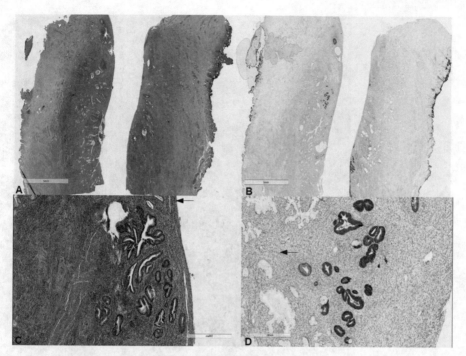

Fig. 6 P16 in endocervical adenocarcinomas. (**a**, **b**) P16 highlights even in this magnification the neoplastic glands in this cone biopsy (**a**, HES ×5; **b**, 5×). (**c**, **d**) It is strongly expressed by neoplastic but not nearby normal glands (**c**, HES ×50; **d**, ×50). *HES* hematoxylin, eosin, safranin. All routine slides presented here are HES-stained. All immunohistochemistry slides are counterstained with hematoxylin

P16 is also useful in distinguishing a vulvar basaloid SCC, which is typically HPV-associated, from a basaloid carcinoma of the vulva, which is p16 negative [24].

In penile lesions, p16 IHC is useful in distinguishing differentiated (simplex) IN from warty/basaloid IN; the first lesion is p16 negative and is associated with invasive SCCs of low grade keratinizing, not associated to HPV, while the latter is p16 positive and is associated with HPV features [25].

Similar to vulva and penis, SCC of the scrotum, in situ or invasive, can be either positive for p16 (almost 40%) which is associated with HPV infection and displays predominantly a basaloid or warty morphology or negative for p16, not-associated with HPV, and of usual-type morphology [26].

3.2.3 Head-and-Neck Cancer

As with cervical neoplasia, interest regarding head-and-neck squamous cell carcinomas (HNSCC) has been regained after the discovery that a proportion of these tumors are HPV-associated with important diagnostic and prognostic consequences. Oropharyngeal carcinomas with a typical nonkeratinizing basaloid morphology and a strong lymphocytic host reaction are usually those associated with HPV infection and they are p16 positive (Fig. 7) [3–5].

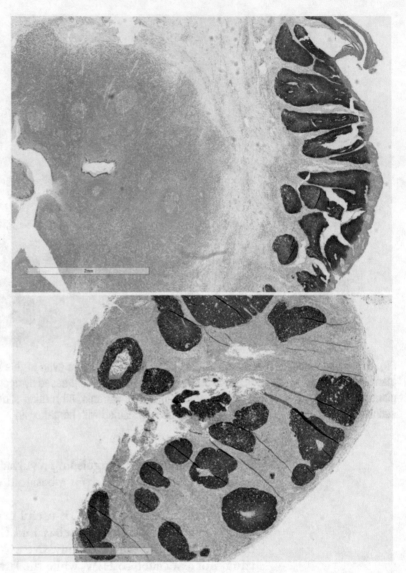

Fig. 7 P16 in head-and-neck squamous cell carcinomas. P16 in tonsillar (**a**, ×20) and oropharyngeal (**b**, ×50) cancer. Strong expression by all tumor cells. All immunohistochemistry slides are counterstained with hematoxylin

HPV-related oropharyngeal squamous cell carcinomas (OPSCCs) represent a distinct entity, as they are associated with sexual risk factors, occur at a younger age, are associated with lower amounts of tobacco use, and have a much better prognosis despite a high propensity for regional lymph node metastases [27]. A constant limitation regarding OPSCC is the algorithm used for HPV detection, as HPV DNA can be detected by PCR but this does not always represent its functional activity, highlighted by the fact that these assays detect HPV even in normal samples, and, on the other hand, using functional dysfunction of HPV targets like p16 IHC may overestimate its prevalence as p16 can be also disrupted by other mechanisms [28]. As such, the HPV detection algorithms proposed, often use multiple assays to detect both the presence of HPV and confirm its functional activity [28]. In these cases, p16 IHC and HPV DNA in situ hybridization (DISH) show a discordance of almost 20%; when using RNA in situ hybridization (RISH), however, for detecting E6/E7 mRNA, an assay that can confirm both the presence of HPV in tumor cells and its transcriptional activity, most (88%) of p16+/HPV DISH− carcinomas are found to harbor transcriptionally active HPV [28]. Thus, in nonkeratinizing or partially nonkeratinizing OPSCCs that are also p16 positive, HPV specific testing is probably unnecessary, as p16 positivity in these tumors imply the presence of transcriptionally active high-risk HPV [27]. Whether HPV-specific testing is necessary for p16-positive keratinizing (or other rare variants) OPSCC remains still controversial, but even among keratinizing OPSCCs p16 and HPV results also correlate well [27].

In oropharyngeal tumors, p16 expression is found in almost 80% of them [27]. Patients with p16 positive tumors have a longer overall survival [29]. Most (80%) p16 positive tumors are HPV positive, whereas the rest of them are HPV negative, a rate that may be ascribed to sample degradation during preparation and storage or to the greater complexity of polymerase chain reaction compared with IHC [29] or it can be really unassociated with HPV [30]. Survival is also better for p16 positive tonsillar and base of the tongue carcinomas [30] and oral carcinomas overexpressing p16 independent of HPV infection [31].

HPV role in non-oropharyngeal SCCs (non-OPSCC) is less well studied. These tumors are p16 positive in almost 20% of the cases [32]. Prognosis for these patients is better than for p16 negative cases, but there is no survival difference when DISH is used for HPV detection [32]. P16 and DISH discordance is almost 15% in these cases [32].

As for the criteria of p16 positivity in HNSCCs, it is recommended to define as p16-positive, cases with >75% p16 positivity or 25–75% positivity but with >75% confluence of positive cells or with >50% p16 positivity with >25% confluence [11]. Also, the proportion of partial staining cases is likely dependent upon the antibody clone utilized, with many of the partial staining cases identified by the clone G175-405, showing clear positivity or negativity when restained with the clone E6H4 [11]. In cytologic material a lower threshold of 10% positive cells, as well as a lower sensitivity of p16 IHC, have been reported [33].

P16 positivity is also frequent (31%) in nodal metastases of cutaneous HNSCC, but this expression has no impact on the clinical outcome neither as a surrogate marker for high-risk HPV subtypes in this context [34]. As such, p16 expression does not always help in the search of an unknown primary [34].

In the rare case of a large cell neuroendocrine carcinoma arising in head/neck regions, HPV can be rarely found, but p16 expression is found in most of these tumors even without HPV infection [35].

3.2.4 Melanocytic Lesions

P16 has a critical role also in melanoma; in most melanomas p16 is disabled by deletion, mutation, or silencing of *CDKN2A*, and germ-line mutations in *CDKN2A* predispose to melanoma with high penetrance [9]. P16 immunohistochemistry has gained attention for the differential diagnosis between benign and malignant melanocytic lesions, as p16 expression is usually present in nevi and absent in melanomas [36]. Similarly, in Spitzoid melanocytic lesions, loss of p16 immunohistochemical expression, corresponding to *CDKN2A* copy loss, is not observed in Spitz nevi (Fig. 8) but it is seen in some borderline atypical Spitzoid tumors (26%) and in some Spitzoid melanomas (16%) [37]. p16 expression loss by dermal melanocytes is also more often seen with melanomas than Spitz tumors [38]. Negative p16 melanomas have adverse tumor features and poorer survival [36].

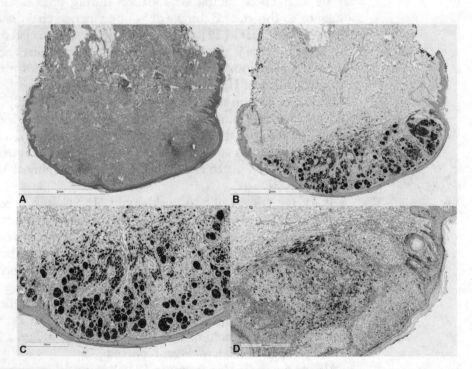

Fig. 8 P16 in melanocytic lesions. (**a–c**) Spitzoid nevus retains p16 expression (**a**, HES ×20; **b**, ×20; **c**, ×50), while a melanoma often loses it (**d**, ×50). In these lesions, alkaline phosphatase is preferred as the chromogen (red) instead of DAB (brown), as they are already brown due to their melanin content. *HES* hematoxylin, eosin, safranin. All routine slides presented here are HES-stained. All immunohistochemistry slides are counterstained with hematoxylin

3.2.5 *Leiomyosarcoma/*
Ovarian and Uterine
Carcinoma

Gene expression studies have demonstrated increased p16 in uterine leiomyosarcoma, an upregulation probably unrelated to human papillomavirus, and this upregulation extends to increased p16 protein expression; several studies have reported increased p16 protein expression in leiomyosarcoma when compared with that in leiomyoma, but this difference is less important when comparing with atypical leiomyoma (leiomyoma with bizarre nuclei) and cellular leiomyoma, the main leiomyoma variants causing diagnostic issues (Fig. 9) [39]. Leiomyoma with bizarre nuclei, a smooth

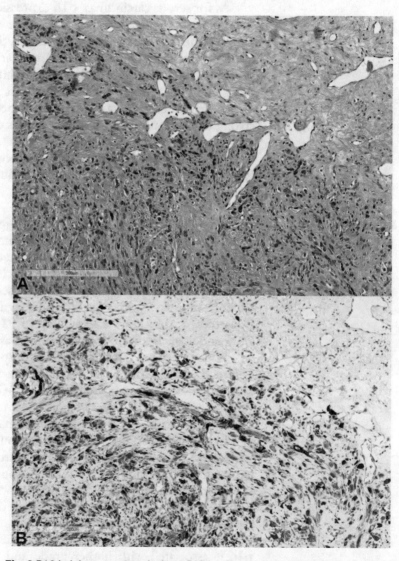

Fig. 9 P16 in leiomyomatous lesions. P16 is often expressed by leiomyomas with bizarre nuclei as in the present lesion (**a**, HES ×100; **b** ×100), as it does with leiomyosarcomas. Thus, its positivity does not help in this differential diagnosis. *HES* hematoxylin, eosin, safranin. All routine slides presented here are HES-stained. All immunohistochemistry slides are counterstained with hematoxylin

muscle tumor with significant atypia but no mitoses or tumor necrosis [40], is probably a benign tumor as most cases described have a benign course [40]; however, rare cases of recurrence have been reported [39]. Moreover, these leiomyomas show the same molecular abnormalities as leiomyosarcomas and as such is not clear if they represent a form of leiomyoma progressing to malignancy or leiomyomas just harboring degenerative cellular features [41]. In any case, p16 or p53 immunohistochemistry is useful when negative, probably excluding a leiomyosarcoma, but it is of no use in this differential diagnosis when positive [42].

As for serous carcinomas, p16 expression is strong and diffuse in contrast to that seen in the lower grade endometrioid adenocarcinoma where there is a patchy expression (Fig. 5). It should always remember that higher grade endometrioid tumors (grade 3) will be also p16 positive. When glandular architecture is found, resembling endometrioid adenocarcinoma, but nuclear atypia is intensive, a serous carcinoma should be suspected. In this case, p16 strong expression is expected with serous carcinoma but not with low grade endometrioid adenocarcinoma. However, in this distinction, p53 immunohistochemical detection is mostly used, as is for establishing the diagnosis of an ovarian/tubal/peritoneal high grade serous carcinoma.

3.2.6   Other Tumors

p16 immunohistochemistry has been suggested for other tumors too, like lipomatous ones. In the differential diagnosis of atypical lipomatous tumor versus well-differentiated liposarcoma p16 positivity has a sensitivity of 89.5% and a specificity of 68.2%, which is impaired by false-positive lipomas with secondary changes, especially in biopsies. In the differential diagnosis of dedifferentiated liposarcoma p16 shows a sensitivity of 94.4% and a specificity of 70%, and as such it is not recommended as a single marker [43].

It may be of use in the distinction of sporadic versus hereditary colorectal carcinomas with microsatellite instability, as p16 IHC might be used as a surrogate marker for *MLH1* promoter methylation; specifically, p16-negative colorectal carcinomas show *MLH1* methylation, whereas hereditary carcinomas are p16-positive [44].

In breast cancer, the 9p21 deletion found in almost 15% of the cases, is associated with adverse tumor features; corresponding p16 expression is lost when there is homozygous 9p21 deletion, though no difference in expression is seen when no deletion or a heterozygous deletion is found [10]. When p16 is overexpressed, as seen in almost 12% of breast carcinomas, adverse tumor features are also observed [10]. Similarly, ductal intraepithelial neoplasia expressing p16 is associated with higher grade and progression to invasive carcinomas [45].

Recently, p16 it has been shown to act as a predictive and prognostic factor for osteosarcomas, where its absence of expression is associated with the absence of response to neoadjuvant chemotherapy and an adverse prognosis [46].

Also, p16 deletion detected by FISH has been emerged as very specific but moderately sensitive method in the distinction of mesothelioma from reactive mesothelial hyperplasia [1].

To conclude, p16 immunohistochemical expression is a useful diagnostic and prognostic marker that can be easily adopted in the routine practice. Caution should be paid regarding its interpretation and indications.

4 Notes

1. Remember to remove excess fluid from the slides in every step with gently draining the slide.

2. Caution with hot objects in steps where high temperature is used.

3. During epitope retrieval, put a metal rack with the slides into appropriate containers containing ER solution and then sink the containers in the deionized water of the pressure cooker. Follow manufacturer's instructions to proceed with boiling.

4. The staining procedure should be carried out in a humid environment as tissue drying will increase nonspecific binding. A simple solution for this would be a plastic box with sealed lid, at the bottom of which a wet paper can be placed. Find a way to level the paper so that the slides lay flat over it.

5. Most commercial kits provide all the above reagents; follow instructions.

6. No or weak staining? Try the following: be sure that the secondary antibody is anti-mouse if your primary is mouse raised, concentrate your primary antibody or incubate longer.

7. High background? Try the following: sections are too thick, sections not well deparaffinized, incubate for a shorter time with ER solution, incubate longer with blocking reagent, dilute the primary antibody or incubate in lower temperature, wash generously with washing buffer, keep sections in humidity.

Acknowledgement

Conflict of interest: The authors have no conflict of interest to disclose.

References

1. Karpathiou G, Stefanou D, Froudarakis ME (2015) Pleural neoplastic pathology. Respir Med 109(8):931–943. https://doi.org/10.1016/j.rmed.2015.05.014

2. Karpathiou G, Da Cruz V, Patoir A et al (2016) Mediastinal cyst of müllerian origin: evidence for developmental endosalpingiosis. Pathology 49(1):83–84

3. Karpathiou G, Casteillo F, Giroult J et al (2016) Prognostic impact of immune microenvironment in laryngeal and pharyngeal squamous cell carcinoma: immune cell subtypes, immunosuppressive pathways and clinicopathologic characteristics. Oncotarget 8(12):19310

4. Karpathiou G, Giroult J, Forest F et al (2016) Clinical and histological predictive factors of response to induction chemotherapy in head and neck squamous cell carcinoma. Am J Clin Pathol 146:546. https://doi.org/10.1093/ajcp/aqw145

5. Karpathiou G, Monaya A, Forest F et al (2016) P16 and p53 expression status in head and neck squamous cell carcinoma: a correlation with histologic, histoprognostic and clinical parameters. Pathology 48(4):341–348

6. Karpathiou G, Sivridis E, Koukourakis MI et al (2011) Light-chain 3A autophagic activity and prognostic significance in non-small cell lung carcinomas. Chest 140(1):127–134

7. Sivridis E, Giatromanolaki A, Karpathiou G, Karpouzis A, Kouskoukis C, Koukourakis MI (2011) LC3A-positive "stone-like" structures in cutaneous squamous cell carcinomas. Am J Dermatopathol 33(3):285–290

8. Karpathiou G, Sivridis E, Koukourakis M et al (2013) Autophagy and Bcl-2/BNIP3 death regulatory pathway in non-small cell lung carcinomas. APMIS 121(7):592–604

9. Karpathiou G, Batistatou A, Forest F, Clemenson A, Peoc'h M (2016) Basic molecular pathology and cytogenetics for practicing pathologists: correlation with morphology and with a focus on aspects of diagnostic or therapeutic utility. Adv Anat Pathol 23(6):368–380

10. Lebok P, Roming M, Kluth M et al (2016) p16 overexpression and 9p21 deletion are linked to unfavorable tumor phenotype in breast cancer. Oncotarget 7(49):81322

11. Barasch S, Mohindra P, Hennrick K, Hartig GK, Harari PM, Yang DT (2016) Assessing p16 status of oropharyngeal squamous cell carcinoma by combined assessment of the number of cells stained and the confluence of p16 staining. Am J Surg Pathol 40(9):1261–1269

12. Kurman R, Carcangiu M, Herrington C, Young R (eds) (2014) WHO classification of tumours of the female reproductive organs, 4th edn. IARC, Lyon

13. Darragh TM, Colgan TJ, Thomas Cox J et al (2013) The lower anogenital squamous terminology standardization project for HPV-associated lesions. Int J Gynecol Pathol 32(1):76–115

14. Thrall M (2016) Effect of lower anogenital squamous terminology recommendations on the use of p16 immunohistochemistry and the proportion of high-grade diagnoses in cervical biopsy specimens. Am J Clin Pathol 145:524–530

15. Maniar KP, Sanchez B, Paintal A, Gursel DB, Nayar R (2015) Role of the biomarker p16 in downgrading -IN 2 diagnoses and predicting higher-grade lesions. Am J Surg Pathol 39(12):1708–1718

16. Pirog EC (2015) Immunohistochemistry and in situ hybridization for the diagnosis and classification of squamous lesions of the anogenital region. Semin Diagn Pathol 32(5):409–418

17. Clark JL, Lu D, Kalir T, Liu Y (2016) Overdiagnosis of HSIL on cervical biopsy: errors in p16 immunohistochemistry implementation. Hum Pathol 55:51–56

18. Lee S, Sabourin J, Gage J, Franko A, Nation J, Duggan M (2015) Squamous intraepithelial lesions in cervical tissue samples of limited adequacy and insufficient for grading as low or high grade: outcome, clinico-pathological correlates, and predictive role of p16INK4a and Ki67 biomarker staining. J Low Genit Tract Dis 19(1):35–45

19. Zhang G, Yang B, Abdul-Karim F (2015) p16 immunohistochemistry is useful in confirming high-grade squamous intraepithelial lesions (HSIL) in women with negative HPV testing. Int J Gynecol Pathol 34:180–186

20. Kusanagi Y, Kojima A, Mikami Y et al (2010) Absence of high-risk human papillomavirus (HPV) detection in endocervical adenocarcinoma with gastric morphology and phenotype. Am J Pathol 177(5):2169–2175

21. Schwartz LE, Khani F, Bishop JA, Vang R, Epstein JI (2016) Carcinoma of the uterine cervix involving the genitourinary tract: a potential diagnostic dilemma. Am J Surg Pathol 40(1):27–35

22. Dong F, Kojiro S, Borger DR, Growdon WB, Oliva E (2015) Squamous cell carcinoma of the vulva. Am J Surg Pathol 39(8):1045–1053

23. Reyes MC, Cooper K (2014) An update on vulvar intraepithelial neoplasia: terminology and a practical approach to diagnosis. J Clin Pathol 67(4):290–294

24. Elwood H, Kim J, Yemelyanova A, Ronnett BM, Taube JM (2014) Basal cell carcinomas of the vulva. Am J Surg Pathol 38(4):542–547

25. Chaux A, Pfannl R, Rodríguez IM et al (2011) Distinctive immunohistochemical profile of penile intraepithelial lesions. Am J Surg Pathol 35(4):553–562

26. Matoso A, Ross HM, Chen S, Allbritton J, Epstein JI (2014) Squamous neoplasia of the scrotum. Am J Surg Pathol 38(7):973–981

27. Gondim DD, Haynes W, Wang X, Chernock RD, El-Mofty SK, Lewis JS (2016) Histologic typing in oropharyngeal squamous cell carcinoma. Am J Surg Pathol 40(8):1117–1124

28. Rooper LM, Gandhi M, Bishop JA, Westra WH (2016) RNA in-situ hybridization is a practical and effective method for determining HPV status of oropharyngeal squamous cell carcinoma including discordant cases that are p16 positive by immunohistochemistry but HPV negative by DNA in-situ hybridization. Oral Oncol 55:11–16

29. Rosenthal DI, Harari PM, Giralt J et al (2016) Association of human papillomavirus and p16 status with outcomes in the IMCL-9815 phase III registration trial for patients with locoregionally advanced oropharyngeal squamous cell carcinoma of the head and neck treated with radiotherapy with or without C. J Clin Oncol 34(12):1300–1308

30. Garnaes E, Frederiksen K, Kiss K et al (2016) Double positivity for HPV DNA/p16 in tonsillar and base of tongue cancer improves prognostication: insights from a large population-based study. Int J Cancer 139(11): 2598–2605

31. Satgunaseelan L, Virk SA, Lum T, Gao K, Clark JR, Gupta R (2016) p16 expression independent of human papillomavirus is associated with lower stage and longer disease-free survival in oral cavity squamous cell carcinoma. Pathology 48(5):441–448

32. Chung CH, Zhang Q, Kong CS et al (2014) p16 protein expression and human papillomavirus status as prognostic biomarkers of nonoropharyngeal head and neck squamous cell carcinoma. J Clin Oncol 32(35):3930–3938

33. Xu B, Ghossein R, Lane J, Lin O, Katabi N (2016) The utility of p16 immunostaining in fine needle aspiration in p16-positive head and neck squamous cell carcinoma. Hum Pathol 54:193–200

34. McDowell LJ, Young RJ, Johnston ML et al (2016) p16-positive lymph node metastases from cutaneous head and neck squamous cell carcinoma: no association with high-risk human papillomavirus or prognosis and implications for the workup of the unknown primary. Cancer 122(8):1201–1208

35. Thompson ED, Stelow EB, Mills SE, Westra WH, Bishop JA (2016) Large cell neuroendocrine carcinoma of the head and neck. Am J Surg Pathol 40(4):471–478

36. Lade-Keller J, Riber-Hansen R, Guldberg P, Schmidt H, Hamilton-Dutoit SJ, Steiniche T (2014) Immunohistochemical analysis of molecular drivers in melanoma identifies p16 as an independent prognostic biomarker. J Clin Pathol 67(6):520–528

37. Harms PW, Hocker TL, Zhao L et al (2016) Loss of p16 expression and copy number changes of CDKN2A in a spectrum of spitzoid melanocytic lesions. Hum Pathol 58:152–160

38. George E, Polissar NL, Wick M (2010) Immunohistochemical evaluation of p16 INK4A, E-cadherin, and cyclin D1 expression in melanoma and spitz tumors. Am J Clin Pathol 133(3):370–379

39. Mills AM, Ly A, Balzer BL et al (2013) Cell cycle regulatory markers in uterine atypical leiomyoma and leiomyosarcoma: immunohistochemical study of 68 cases with clinical follow-up. Am J Surg Pathol 37(5):634–642

40. Croce S, Young R, Oliva E (2014) Uterine leiomyomas with bizarre nuclei A clinicopathologic study of 59 cases. Am J Surg Pathol 38(10):1330–1339

41. Liegl-Atzwanger B, Heitzer E, Flicker K et al (2016) Exploring chromosomal abnormalities and genetic changes in uterine smooth muscle tumors. Mod Pathol 29(10):1262–1277

42. Oliva E (2016) Practical issues in uterine pathology from banal to bewildering: the remarkable spectrum of smooth muscle neoplasia. Mod Pathol 29:S104–S120

43. Kammerer-Jacquet S, Sixte T, Cabilic F et al (2017) Differential diagnosis of atypical lipomatous tumor/well-differentiated liposarcoma and dedifferentiated liposarcoma: utility of p16 in combination with MDM2 and CDK4 immunohistochemistry. Hum Pathol 59:34–40

44. Boissière-Michot F, Frugier H, Ho-Pun-Cheung A, Lopez-Crapez E, Duffour J, Bibeau F (2016) Immunohistochemical staining for p16 and BRAFV600E is useful to distinguish between sporadic and hereditary (Lynch syndrome-related) microsatellite instable colorectal carcinomas. Virchows Arch 469(2):135–144

45. Bechert C, Kim J-Y, Tramm T, Tavassoli FA (2016) Co-expression of p16 and p53 characterizes aggressive subtypes of ductal intraepithelial neoplasia. Virchows Arch 469(6): 659–667

46. Righi A, Gambarotti M, Sbaraglia M et al (2016) p16 expression as a prognostic and predictive marker in high-grade localized osteosarcoma of the extremities: an analysis of 357 cases. Hum Pathol 58:15–23

Chapter 13

Detection of E2F-DNA Complexes Using Chromatin Immunoprecipitation Assays

Miyoung Lee, Lorraine J. Gudas, and Harold I. Saavedra

Abstract

Chromatin immunoprecipitation (ChIP), originally developed by John T. Lis and David Gilmour in 1984, has been useful to detect DNA sequences where protein(s) of interest bind. ChIP is comprised of several steps: (1) cross-linking of proteins to target DNA sequences, (2) breaking genomic DNA into 300–1000 bp pieces by sonication or nuclease digestion, (3) immunoprecipitation of protein bound to target DNA with an antibody, (4) reverse cross-linking between target DNA and the bound protein to liberate the DNA fragments, and (5) amplification of target DNA fragment by PCR. Since then, the technology has evolved significantly to allow not only amplifying target sequences by PCR, but also sequencing all DNA fragment bound to a target protein, using a variant of the approach called the ChIP-seq technique (1). Another variation, the ChIP-on-ChIP, allows the detection of protein complexes bound to specific DNA sequences (2).

Key words Chromatin immunoprecipitation (ChIP), E2Fs, Nek2 promoter, Plk4 promoter, Her2+ breast cancer cell lines

1 Introduction

Chromatin immunoprecipitation (ChIP) was originally developed by John T. Lis and David Gilmour in 1984, in order to test the binding of RNA polymerase from *E. coli* to a constitutively expressed, *lambda cI* gene, and to the isopropyl beta-D-thiogalactoside (IPTG) uninduced and induced *lac* operon [1]. They tested this method in vivo by detecting the binding of RNA polymerase II-DNA interactions in untreated or heat-shocked *Drosophila melanogaster* cells, where they demonstrated that binding of this protein increased at specific DNA sequences in response to heat shock [2]. Since then, it has been heavily used to identify DNA sequences where target proteins, mostly transcription factors, bind to regulate transcription.

ChIP is comprised of several steps: (1) cross-linking proteins to target DNA sequences, (2) breaking genomic DNA into

Pedro G. Santiago-Cardona (ed.), *The Retinoblastoma Protein*, Methods in Molecular Biology, vol. 1726,
https://doi.org/10.1007/978-1-4939-7565-5_13, © Springer Science+Business Media, LLC 2018

300–1000 bp pieces by sonication or nuclease digestion, (3) immunoprecipitation of protein bound to target DNA with antibody, (4) reverse cross-linking between target DNA and a protein to liberate the DNA fragment, and (5) amplification of target DNA fragment by PCR. The technology has evolved significantly, and it now allows not only the amplification of target sequences by PCR, but also sequencing all DNA fragment bound to a specific target protein, in a variation of the approach called the ChIP-seq technique [3]. Another variation, the ChIP-on-ChIP, allows the detection of protein complexes bound to specific DNA sequences [4].

ChIP and its variations have been used to identify novel targets of the transcription factor family collectively called E2Fs. For example, Dynlacht et al. used this powerful technique in combination with DNA sequencing to identify transcripts directly regulated by the E2F transcription factors in human cells [5]. These genes included previously identified genes involved in canonical functions of the E2Fs, such as DNA replication, but also previously unidentified target genes involved in other processes, including mitosis, chromosome condensation and segregation, DNA damage checkpoints, and DNA repair. This work was critical to the Rb/E2F field, since it suggested that E2Fs could regulate several important cellular functions besides the control of S phase. For example, their RT-PCR analyses identified elevated levels of the mitotic and spindle assembly checkpoint regulators TTK, Mad2L, Hec1, and Nek2 in mouse embryonic fibroblasts lacking the Rb family members p130 and p107, which antagonize E2F function. Farnham et al. used ChIP to identify novel E2F promoters with consensus, and nonconsensus E2F sequences [6], and combined Chip with a CpG array to show that E2Fs bound nonconsensus sites to regulate expression of genes that are involved in recombination and DNA repair [7]. Nevins et al. used ChIP to show that E2Fs transcription factors coordinate G1/S and G2/M by differential binding of E2F repressors (E2F4) and activators (E2F1, E2F2 and E2F3) to negative or positive E2F sites within promoters of genes that are involved in mitotic entry and exit, including cdc2 [8].

Our laboratory has used ChIP to show that E2F1, E2F2, and E2F3 bind the promoters of the centrosome and mitotic regulators Nek2 and Plk4 to regulate their expression [9]. We uncovered these findings by adapting a protocol from The Gudas lab [10]. We also found that the E2Fs were sufficient to induce centrosome amplification and chromosome instability in mammary epithelial and breast cancer cells in part by maintaining high levels of Nek2. An unpublished example of how the E2F activators E2F1, E2F2, and E2F3 bind to the Plk4 promoter in Her2$^+$ JIMT-1 and SKBR3 breast cancer cells is presented in Fig. 1. This figure also shows the limitation of shRNA-mediated knockdown and ChIP, since, while

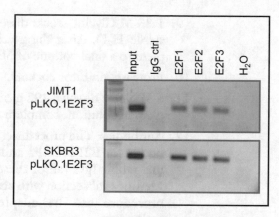

Fig. 1 ChIP on putative E2F binding site on Plk4 promoter. Immunoprecipitation (IP) was performed on two Her2+ breast cancer cell lines, JIMT1 and SKBR3 knocked down for E2F3 using E2F1, E2F2, or E2F3 antibody. Control IgG was used as a negative control for IP. Then, PCR was performed with primer set that covers tentative E2F binding sites on Plk4 promoter region. Input was used as a positive control for PCR

E2F3 occupancy on the promoter was clearly reduced relative to input, there was still some E2F3 bound to the promoter. While shRNA-mediated knockdown results in reduced protein levels, there is always some left, and that is why technologies that have achieved complete knockdown of proteins, including Cas9/CRISPR have emerged [11, 12]. Also, the presence of E2F3 on the promoter may also reflect the inability of E2F3 protein to be degraded upon binding to a promoter.

2 Materials

2.1 Reagents and Solutions

1. RIPA buffer: 50 mM Tris–HCl (pH 8.0), 150 mM NaCl, 5 mM EDTA, 1% NP-40, 0.5% sodium deoxycholate, 0.1% SDS (*see* **Note 1**).

2. ChIP wash buffer: 50 mM Tris–HCl (pH 8.5), 500 mM LiCl, 1% NP-40, 1% sodium deoxycholate.

3. TE buffer: 10 mM Tris–HCl (pH 8.0), 1 mM EDTA (pH 8.0).

4. ChIP elution buffer: 50 mM Tris–HCl (pH 8.0), 1% SDS, 1 mM EDTA (pH 8.0).

5. Protein A Sepharose.

6. Qiagen QIAquick PCR Purification Kit (Cat. No. 28106).

7. $1\times$ Phosphate Buffered Saline (PBS): 137 mM NaCl, 2.7 mM KCl, 10 mM Na_2HPO_4, 2 mM KH_2PO_4 (pH 7.4).

8. Formaldehyde 37%.

9. 1.25 M Glycine stock: dissolve 46.92 g of glycine in 400 mL sterile H_2O. After the glycine is completely dissolved, complete to a final volume of 500 mL with sterile H_2O.

10. Protease inhibitor cocktail.

11. 5 M NaCl: dissolve 292 g of NaCl in 800 mL H_2O, after complete dissolution, complete to 1 L final volume with H_2O.

12. Antibodies: The procedures described in this chapter use antibodies for E2F1, E2F2 and E2F3 as well as nonimmune normal rabbit IgG (all of these are described in the appropriate Methods subsection with accompanying notes). However, this procedure can be adapted to work with a variety of antibodies.

13. Cell lines: We have successfully applied the ChIP protocol in this chapter to JIMT1 (breast carcinoma) and SKBR3 (breast adenocarcinoma) cell lines, but the procedure described below can be adapted for any cell line. Our cell lines are described below in the appropriate Methods subsection. Culture your cell lines in culture media and conditions appropriate for them, and follow the guidelines described in Subheading 3 below regarding the cell density and percent of confluence recommended for the procedure.

14. Goat anti-mouse IgM.

15. Primer sets: according to target sequence of interest.

2.2 Equipment and Labware

1. Orbital shaker.

2. Cell scrapers.

3. 15 mL tubes.

4. Probe sonicator.

5. 1.5 mL microcentrifuge tubes.

6. Heat block.

3 Methods

In preparation, and before starting the procedure, you need to plate ~2.5×10^6 cells in p150 mm culture dishes for each treatment or group. Culture medium depends on the cell type. In this protocol, we used JIMT1 (breast carcinoma) and SKBR3 (breast adenocarcinoma) cell lines. We cultured the parental cell lines, as well as their derivatives expressing empty vector -PLKO.1-, or stably knocked down for E2F3 by lentiviral mediated transduction (as a negative control in our experiments). We keep JIMT1 cells in DMEM with 10% FBS, 1× Penicillin/Streptomycin, with 2 µg/mL puromycin, while we keep SKBR3 in RPMI1640 with 10% FBS,

1× Penicillin/Streptomycin, with 2 µg/mL puromycin. However, it must be noticed that the procedure described below is applicable to a great variety of cell lines. You must culture cells until they reach confluence.

3.1 Chromatin Preparation and Antibody Binding to Cross-Linked Chromatin (Day 1)

1. To start your experiments, be sure to have at least 2×10^7 cells in your cultures at the time of harvest (this should be about 80–90% confluence). You test this by setting a pilot experiment where you plate various numbers of cells and harvest cells for counting when they become confluent.

2. Add formaldehyde (37% solution) to a final concentration 1% directly to the media (540 µL in 20 mL media) to cross-link cells, and put plates on shaker and shake vigorously for 10 min at room temperature.

3. Add glycine to a final concentration of 0.15 M to quench the cross-linking reaction, and incubate on shaker for at least 5 min at room temperature.

4. Discard media from plates and wash cells with ~10 mL cold 1× PBS twice.

5. Add 1–2 mL of cold 1× PBS to each plate, scrape cells off the plate, and transfer cells to a labeled 15 mL tube stored on ice.

6. Centrifuge cells for 5 min at 4 °C at $5000 \times g$.

7. Discard supernatant by aspiration, suspend pellet in 350 µL of RIPA buffer containing protease inhibitors by gently pipetting pellet up and down, and transfer to labeled prechilled 1.5 mL microcentrifuge tube on ice (*see* **Note 2**).

8. Sonicate samples for 15 s using a probe sonicator. Choose the sonicator setting such that the output should be ~6–7 amp. Keep samples on ice after sonication and repeat sonication one more time (*see* **Note 3**).

9. Harvest sonicated samples by centrifuging for 10 min at 4 °C at $12,000 \times g$ (*see* **Note 4**).

10. Transfer soluble supernatant which should contain the chromatin to a clean 1.5 mL microcentrifuge tube and adjust the volume to 50 µL with RIPA buffer, so each tube contains material from an estimated $3–3.5 \times 10^6$ cells. Each of these tubes will be used in an immunoprecipitation (IP) reaction in subsequent steps.

11. To make one IP reaction, to the 50 µL volume from **step 10**, add 450 µL of RIPA buffer with protease inhibitors (*see* **Note 5**).

12. To preclear the chromatin-containing soluble supernatant, add 75 µL of 50% Protein A sepharose/1× PBS (v:v) slurry in each reaction tube and incubate on a rocker at 4 °C for 15 min to several hours (*see* **Note 6**).

13. Spin down the precleared chromatin by centrifuging at $3000 \times g$ for 30 s.

14. Transfer 475 μL of precleared soluble chromatin to a clean microcentrifuge tube. Save extra precleared soluble chromatin for input control during PCR.

15. Add 2 μg antibody of interest to each immunoprecipitation (IP) tube and incubate at 4 °C overnight on shaker. For our particular purpose, we used antibodies against E2F1, E2F2, and E2F3. Set a negative control by using normal nonimmune rabbit IgG (*see* **Notes 7–9**).

3.2 Immuno-precipitation and Reversion of Cross-Link (Day 2)

1. Spin down each IP tube by brief centrifugation, add 50 μL of 50% Protein A slurry to each tube, and incubate for 1 h on a rocker at 4 °C. When using monoclonal antibodies, add 2.5 μg of goat anti-mouse IgM to each tube and incubate 1 h before adding Protein A Sepharose slurry).

2. Centrifuge tubes at $3000 \times g$ for 30 s and discard supernatant by aspiration.

3. To wash pellet, add 1 mL of RIPA buffer, and incubate on rocker for 5 min at room temperature and spin down at $3000 \times g$ for 30 s.

4. Repeat **step 3** one more time.

5. Wash pellet twice with ChIP wash buffer.

6. Wash pellet with TE buffer twice and after second wash, remove supernatant as much as possible.

7. Add 100 μL of ChIP elution buffer to each IP tube. Elution buffer should be made fresh and used within a month after preparation.

8. Incubate at 65 °C in a heat block for 10 min.

9. Vortex all samples for 15 s and spin down samples at $12,000 \times g$ for 30 s (*see* **Note 10**).

10. Transfer 100 μL of supernatant to a new tube containing 4 μL of 5 M NaCl and reverse the cross-linking by incubating samples at 65 °C in a heat block overnight. Set up an input control tube by adding 75 μL of elution buffer containing 5 μL of 5 M NaCl per 25 μL of precleared soluble chromatin.

3.3 DNA Isolation and PCR Amplification of Target Sequence (Day 3)

To isolate DNA fragments, we use Qiagen QIAquick PCR purification kit (Cat. No. 28106, Qiagen), following manufacturer's instructions.

1. Remove tubes from heat block and spin down condensation.

2. Add 500 μL of PB buffer from the Qiagen kit to each tube and vortex it for a couple minutes.

Table 1
Primers used in ChIP for Nek2 and Plk4 target genes

	Sequences
Nek2_F	5′-TTG GCG ATC TCT ATC AGA GGG-3′
Nek_R	5′-AAA GTG TCA CTA GGC AAC CGC-3′
Plk4_F	5′-AGT GTC CCG AGG CAC TGC GGC TT-3′
Plk4_R	5′-AGA TAA CCG CCA TCC CCT TGG A-3′

3. Spin down for 30 s at $12,000 \times g$.

4. Transfer solution to Qiagen column and centrifuge for 1 min at $12,000 \times g$.

5. Discard flow-through and wash column with 750 μL of Qiagen PE wash buffer.

6. Spin down for 30 s at $12,000 \times g$ and discard flow-through.

7. Remove any residual wash buffer by centrifuging tube for an additional 1 min.

8. Remove the Qiagen column and place it a new microcentrifuge tube.

9. Add 50 μL of the kit's elution buffer to the center of column and centrifuge for 1 min at $12,000 \times g$ to collect DNA fragments.

10. Use this for semiquantitative or real-time PCR. *See* Table 1 for the primers that we used for our particular target genes [9].

11. Evaluate results by loading the PCR product in a 2% agarose gel. Figure 1 depicts a typical result from a ChIP experiment, in this case, for the target genes of our interest.

4 Notes

1. Adding SDS is optional since some antibodies may not be compatible with SDS.

2. We used complete mini protease inhibitor cocktail (Cat. No. 11 836 153 001) from Roche. It comes in the form of a tablet and we add 1 tablet/10 mL lysis buffer.

3. It most likely happens that samples can be overheated or overflowed during sonication. You can avoid or minimize these possibilities by either not putting the sonicator at the surface of the samples or by sonicating samples on ice.

4. You will see slightly black debris pellet at the bottom after centrifugation, which is expected and normal.

5. You need to set-up at least two IPs, one for Ab of your interest and one for negative control. To make multiple IP reactions, for example 3 IPs, add 150 μL of chromatin from **step 10** into 1350 μL of RIPA buffer containing protease inhibitor.

6. We used protein Sepharose CL-4b from GE Healthcare life science (cat#17-0780-01) and prepared slurry following manufacturer's guide (according to the manual, 1 g of protein Sepharose CL-4b powder usually generates 4–5 mL of slurry after swelling).

7. The amount of antibody needs to be optimized. Generally speaking, you need to add more if you use polyclonal antibody compared to monoclonal antibody. When you test an antibody for the first time in a ChIP protocol, it is better to include an antibody previously tested in your laboratory and shown to work in your hands.

8. This protocol was performed with the following antibodies: E2F1, Cat. No. 3742, Cell Signaling; E2F2, c-633; Santa Cruz Biotechnology; and E2F3, Cat. No. sc-878, Santa-Cruz biotechnology. However, a standard ChIP protocol such as the one described here can be adapted to a variety of antibodies.

9. Normal rabbit IgG, we use Cell Signaling Cat. No. 2729.

10. Vortex speed sets up between 5 and 7 to avoid breaking the interactions between the antibody and DNA.

Acknowledgments

This research project was supported by PSM-2U54 CA163071-06 and MCC-2U54 CA163068-06 from the National Institutes of Health. The project was also supported by 2U54MD007587 from the PRCTRC, G12MD007579 from RCMI, 4R25GM082406-10 from RISE, The Puerto Rico Science, Technology and Research Trust, and Ponce Medical School Foundation Inc. under the cooperative agreement 2016-00026. The content is solely the responsibility of the authors and does not necessarily represent the official views of the National Institutes of Health.

References

1. Gilmour DS, Lis JT (1984) Detecting protein-DNA interactions in vivo: distribution of RNA polymerase on specific bacterial genes. Proc Natl Acad Sci U S A 81(14):4275–4279

2. Gilmour DS, Lis JT (1985) In vivo interactions of RNA polymerase II with genes of Drosophila melanogaster. Mol Cell Biol 5(8):2009–2018

3. Johnson DS, Mortazavi A, Myers RM, Wold B (2007) Genome-wide mapping of in vivo protein-DNA interactions. Science 316(5830):1497–1502

4. Aparicio O, Geisberg JV, Struhl K (2004) Chromatin immunoprecipitation for determining the association of proteins with specific genomic sequences in vivo. Curr Protoc Cell Biol. Chapter 17: Unit 17. 7

5. Ren BCH, Takahashi Y, Volkert T, Terragni J, Young RA, Dynlacht BD (2002) E2F integrates cell cycle progression with DNA repair, replication, and G(2)/M checkpoints. Genes Dev 16(2):245–256

6. Weinmann AS, Bartley SM, Zhang T, Zhang MQ, Farnham PJ (2001) Use of chromatin immunoprecipitation to clone novel E2F target promoters. Mol Cell Biol 21(20): 6820–6832

7. Weinmann AS, Yan PS, Oberley MJ, Huang TH, Farnham PJ (2002) Isolating human transcription factor targets by coupling chromatin immunoprecipitation and CpG island microarray analysis. Genes Dev 16(2): 235–244

8. Zhu W, Giangrande PH, Nevins JR (2004) E2Fs link the control of G1/S and G2/M transcription. EMBO J 23(23):4615–4626

9. Lee MY, Moreno CS, Saavedra HI (2014) The E2F activators signal and maintain centrosome amplification in breast cancer cells. Mol Cell Biol 34(14):2581–2599

10. Gillespie RF, Gudas LJ (2007) Retinoid regulated association of transcriptional co-regulators and the polycomb group protein SUZ12 with the retinoic acid response elements of Hoxa1, RARbeta(2), and Cyp26A1 in F9 embryonal carcinoma cells. J Mol Biol 372(2):298–316

11. Munoz IM, Szyniarowski P, Toth R, Rouse J, Lachaud C (2014) Improved genome editing in human cell lines using the CRISPR method. PLoS One 9(10):e109752

12. Ma M, Ye AY, Zheng W, Kong L (2013) A guide RNA sequence design platform for the CRISPR/Cas9 system for model organism genomes. Biomed Res Int 2013:270805

Detection of E2F-Induced Transcriptional Activity Using a Dual Luciferase Reporter Assay

Ainhoa Iglesias-Ara, Nerea Osinalde, and Ana M. Zubiaga

Abstract

The E2F transcription factors are key targets for the retinoblastoma (RB) tumor suppressor function. The active or inactive status of RB determines the degree by which E2F-dependent gene expression will occur in a given condition. Changes in transcriptional activity in response to extracellular or intracellular stimuli are frequently measured using genetic reporter assays. In particular, dual luciferase reporter assays are most recommended for this purpose because of their improved experimental accuracy. Here we illustrate the usefulness of the dual luciferase reporter assay to detect E2F-mediated transcriptional activity upon overexpression of E2F1 in cultured cells as readout for RB status and function.

Key words Dual luciferase assay, E2F transcription factors, RB pathway, Transcriptional regulation, Promoters, Transfection

1 Introduction

The Retinoblastoma (RB) family members (p105/pRB, p107, p130) are key components of the RB pathway that play a central role in cell proliferation and cell death via modulation of gene expression. RB lacks intrinsic DNA-binding activity but is recruited to specific genomic locations through interactions with the E2F transcription factors (E2F1-5) [1]. Mammalian E2F transcription factors regulate many genes whose products drive cell cycle progression by binding to the TTTCCCGC consensus motif present in the promoters of these genes [2]. Biochemical studies have shown that E2F's transcriptional activity is determined by the phosphorylation status of RB [2]. Hypophosphorylated RB associates with E2F at the promoter of target genes in resting nonproliferative cells, thereby preventing it from interacting with the cell's transcription machinery and repressing gene expression. Upon cell cycle entry, cyclin/CDK complex-mediated phosphorylations inactivate RB. Consequently, free E2F is able to induce transcriptional activation of its target genes, facilitating G1–S transition,

Pedro G. Santiago-Cardona (ed.), *The Retinoblastoma Protein*, Methods in Molecular Biology, vol. 1726,
https://doi.org/10.1007/978-1-4939-7565-5_14, © Springer Science+Business Media, LLC 2018

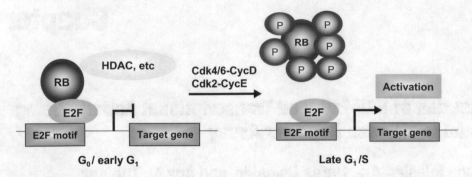

Fig. 1 Model for the regulatory mechanism of E2F transcription factor by the RB pathway. When hypophosphorylated, active RB is bound to E2F, thus blocking E2F transactivation function and inhibiting cell cycle progression. During cell cycle transition from G1 to S phase, cyclin/CDK complexes phosphorylate RB, which leads to free E2F, increased target gene expression and cell cycle progression

DNA replication, and S-phase progression (Fig. 1). Importantly, most tumor cells harbor mutations in components of the RB pathway leading to functional inactivation of RB and aberrant activation of E2F [1]. Thus, E2F activity is tightly linked to RB status, and experimental approaches focusing on E2F-mediated transcriptional activity are commonly used as readout to assess RB function.

Changes in gene transcription can be easily monitored with the use of reporter plasmids (pGL-based vectors) carrying a promoter element of interest fused to a reporter gene, typically luciferase gene from the firefly beetle (*Photinus pyralis*) [3]. When expressed, firefly luciferase converts its substrate D-luciferin into oxyluciferin and emits a specific light signal at 560 nm that can be detected with a luminometer (Fig. 2). The magnitude of the activity corresponding to the reporter protein is usually directly proportional to its transcription level. The efficiency, sensitivity and wide dynamic range of luciferase have made it the preferred choice for assays focusing on gene transcription. To study transcriptional regulation a series of promoter deletion fragments are usually cloned into the pGL vector and tested for luciferase activity to identify specific DNA sequences that mediate transactivation [4–7]. These individual motifs can be further characterized by fine mutational analysis in reporter assays. Luciferase reporter systems have been used extensively to examine gene regulation by RB/E2F, resulting in the identification and fine mapping of many RB/E2F-specific gene promoters [5, 8–10].

A particularly useful tool to assess the mechanisms of RB/E2F-mediated transcriptional regulation in cells relies on the use of reporter constructs carrying synthetic promoters. For these studies, one or multiple copies of the canonical E2F binding motif are inserted immediately upstream of a heterologous basal promoter in

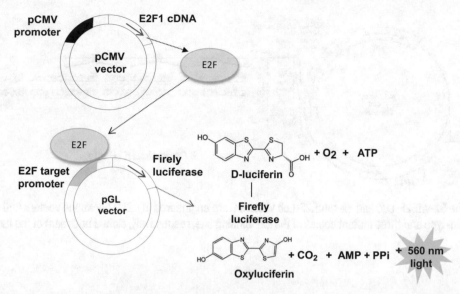

Fig. 2 Components of the dual luciferase reporter system assay. Upon cotransfection of pRc-CMV-E2F1, a plasmid that constitutively expresses human E2F1, with a pGL vector carrying an E2F target promoter cloned immediately upstream of luciferase gene, luciferase activity is induced

the pGL backbone, to generate reporter vectors containing synthetic E2F promoters (Fig. 3). To control for the specificity of E2F-dependent transcriptional activity, synthetic promoters carrying mutated E2F sites are generated in parallel (Fig. 3). By cotransfecting synthetic reporter plasmids along with plasmids driving the expression of E2F protein a significant luciferase activity can be detected in cells carrying wild-type E2F motifs, but not in cells carrying mutant E2F motifs (Fig. 4). This straightforward experimental setting allows assessing efficiently the impact of RB/E2F pathway modulators on transcriptional regulation [10, 11].

Cells are inherently complex, and the data available from a single reporter may be insufficient to differentiate genetic responses of interest from nonrelevant influences in the experimental system. To improve experimental accuracy, dual reporter assays are frequently used. This approach, based on simultaneous use of two independent reporter systems, minimizes experimental variability caused by differences in cell viability, transfection, or cell lysis efficiency. The second reporter acts independently of the experimental conditions and serves as an internal control to normalize data generated by the experimental reporter. The *Renilla* luciferase form the sea pansy (*Renilla reniformis*) is typically used as control reporter, cloned in pRL-TK vectors to provide low to moderate constitutive protein expression. *Renilla* luciferase catalyzes a chemical reaction generating coelenteramide and a specific light signal with a peak emission at 480 nm (Fig. 5). Thus, normalizing the activity of firefly luciferase to the activity of *Renilla* luciferase, transcriptional potential of the cloned regulatory sequence can be

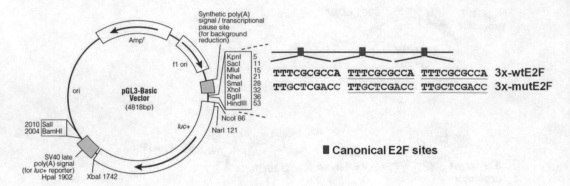

Fig. 3 The 3x-wtE2F-Luc and 3x-mutE2F-Luc vectors were engineered in pGL3 backbone vectors and contain three wild-type and three mutant copies of the E2F binding site, respectively, cloned upstream of the luciferase gene

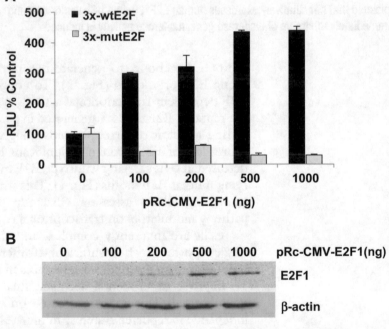

Fig. 4 E2F1 induces gene transcription through canonical E2F binding motifs (3x-wtE2F-Luc), but not through mutated E2F motifs (3x-mutE2F-Luc). (**a**) HEK293T cells were transfected with the indicated luciferase reporter constructs and increasing amounts of pRc-CMV-E2F1 ranging from 100 to 1000 ng. A plasmid expressing *Renilla* luciferase was cotransfected to normalize luciferase activity accounting for transfection efficiency. Relative luciferase activity (RLU) is presented as a ratio of firefly/*Renilla* intensities. Data are shown as percentage over the empty pRc-CMV transfection. The values shown represent the mean±SD ($n = 3$ replicates). (**b**) Western blot analysis of protein extracts demonstrates efficient transfection and dose-dependent expression of pRc-CMV-E2F1 vector in all the experimental conditions

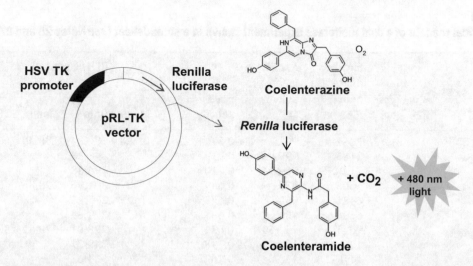

Fig. 5 Components of the dual luciferase reporter system assay. In the experimental setting, a pRL vector that constitutively expresses *Renilla* is also cotransfected and the signal arising from its activity is used to control for nonrelevant effects in the experimental system

inferred [12] (Table 1, Fig. 4). In this chapter, we illustrate the suitability of the dual luciferase reporter assay to study RB/E2F-dependent transcriptional regulation. Particularly, we show that E2F-induced transcriptional activity after expression of E2F1 in cultured cells relies on the presence of consensus E2F binding motifs.

2 Materials

Prepare all solutions using ultrapure water.

2.1 Cell Culture

1. Human embryonic kidney (HEK) 293T cells (*see* **Note 1**).

2. Cell culture media: Dulbecco's modified Eagle's medium (DMEM) supplemented with 10% FBS (*see* **Note 2**).

3. Phosphate-buffered saline (PBS) solution for cell washing. To prepare 10× PBS weigh 25.6 g $Na_2HPO_4 \cdot 7H_2O$, 2 g KCl, and 2 g KH_2PO_4. Add water to a volume of 1 L. Autoclave for 40 min at 121 °C. Store at room temperature.

4. Gibco™ Trypsin–EDTA (0.25%) Phenol Red Solution Thermo-Fisher Scientific. Store at 4 °C (*see* **Note 3**).

5. 0.4% Trypan Blue in PBS. Store at 4 °C (*see* **Note 4**).

6. Hemocytometer or Neubauer chamber and coverslip (*see* **Note 5**).

Table 1
Numerical readout of a dual luciferase experiment shown in a spreadsheet (*see* Notes 26 and 27)

	pRc- CMV-E2F1 (ng)	Firefly luciferase activity (560 nm)	*Renilla* luciferase activity (480 nm)	Firefly/*Renilla* activity	Mean	RLU % control Data	Mean	SD
3x-wtE2F LUC	0	2232	9075	0.246	0.228	107.84	100.00	6.79
		2185	9992	0.219		95.88		
		21,005	95,664	0.220		96.28		
	100	6605	9591	0.689		301.96	298.86	3.37
		6435	9556	0.673		295.27		
		6530	9565	0.683		299.34		
	200	9041	14,259	0.634		278.01	320.82	37.83
		12,472	15,635	0.798		349.77		
		11,452	15,004	0.763		334.67		
	500	10,728	10,887	0.985		432.07	436.45	4.54
		10,620	10,556	1.006		441.13		
		10,708	10,765	0.995		436.15		
	1000	9016	8718	1.034		453.46	441.22	12.60
		9215	9434	0.977		428.29		
		9132	9061	1.008		441.91		
3x-mutE2F LUC	0	187	10,455	0.018	0.021	83.54	100.00	20.53
		255	9682	0.026		123.01		
		201	10,045	0.020		93.46		
	100	110	12,939	0.009		39.71	41.82	1.84
		97	10,584	0.009		42.80		
		104	11,306	0.009		42.96		
	200	146	11,629	0.013		58.64	62.09	3.13
		178	12,839	0.014		64.75		
		154	11,436	0.013		62.89		
	500	53	10,424	0.005		23.75	30.04	6.70
		82	10,326	0.008		37.09		
		63	10,045	0.006		29.29		
	1000	33	5801	0.006		26.57	30.12	3.11
		57	8225	0.007		32.37		
		46	6835	0.007		31.43		

2.2 Transfection

1. Vectors: pRc-CMV, pRc-CMV-E2F1, pGL3-3x-wtE2F, pGL3-3x-mutE2F, and pRL-TK (*see* **Note 6** and Figs. 2, 3, and 5).

2. XtremeGENE HD (Roche) (*see* **Note 7**).

3. Gibco™ Opti-MEM™: Reduced-Serum Medium, an improved Minimal Essential Medium (MEM) that allows for a reduction of Fetal Bovine Serum supplementation (*see* **Note 8**).

2.3 Preparation of Cell Extracts

1. Passive lysis buffer (PLB) of Dual-Luciferase® Reporter Assay System, Promega #E1960. Add 4 volumes of distilled water to 1 volume of 5× PLB to produce 1× PLB (*see* **Note 9**).

2. Plate rocker (Heidolph 36130180 Unimax 1010 Orbital Platform Shaker).

3. Microcentrifuge tubes.

2.4 Determination/ Measurement of Luciferase Activities

1. Luciferase assay reagent (LAR II). Resuspend the lyophilized Luciferase Assay Substrate of Dual-Luciferase® Reporter Assay System, Promega #E1960 in 10 mL of the supplied Luciferase Assay Buffer II (*see* **Note 10**).

2. Stop & Glo® Reagent. Dilute the Stop & Glo® Substrate 50× using the Stop & Glo® buffer provided by the Dual-Luciferase® Reporter Assay System, Promega #E1960 (*see* **Note 11**).

3. Dual injector system Clarity™ Luminescence Microplate Reader (BioTek) (*see* **Note 12**).

3 Methods

3.1 Cell Culture

1. 293T cells are cultured and maintained in DMEM media supplemented with 10% FBS. The cell culture is maintained at 37 °C in a humidified atmosphere of 5% CO_2 in air (*see* **Note 13**).

2. When cell confluence reaches maximum (80–90%), proceed to split cells (*see* **Note 14**). First, rinse cell monolayer twice with 1× PBS. Add prewarmed 0.05% Trypsin–EDTA solution and incubate at 37 °C for 5 min (*see* **Note 15**). Once cell layer is dispersed deactivate trypsin by adding complete growth medium with 10% FBS. Place cell suspension in a new tube.

3. Dilute a minor fraction of cell suspension in 0.4% Trypan Blue and incubate for 2 min at room temperature (*see* **Note 16**).

4. Estimate cell concentration using the hemocytometer and the following formula (*see* **Note 17**).

Total cells/mL = Total cell counted × (dilution factor/# of squares in hemocytometer) × 10,000 cell/mL

5. Dilute cells using complete culture media so that concentration is 1.25×10^5 cell/mL and place 2 mL (2.5×10^5 cells) in each well of 6-well culture plates (*see* **Note 18**).

6. Keep cells growing in an incubator for 24 h at 37 °C in a humidified atmosphere of 5% CO_2.

3.2 Transfections

1. For each experimental condition prepare the corresponding transfection mix containing the plasmid DNA (Table 2): 200 ng of target pGL3 plasmid (firefly) and 20 ng of pRL-TK control vector (*Renilla*) are added to all the mixes (*see* **Note 19**). Additionally, increasing amounts of pRc-CMV-E2F1 vector can be added to the mixes. pRc-CMV empty

vector is supplemented to have a total amount of 2 μg plasmid DNA in all the mixes (Table 1) (*see* **Note 20**).

2. Add the plasmid DNA to 100 μL Opti-MEM for each well and mix it gently by inverting the tube. Next add 2.5 μL XtremeGENE HP (*see* **Note 21**) to the mixture, mix gently, and incubate at room temperature for 25 min (transfection solution).

3. Add the transfection solution to the cells drop-wise and incubate for 24 h (*see* **Note 22**).

3.3 Preparation of Cell Extracts

1. Remove the medium from the cells to be assayed. Wash the cells once with 1× PBS and add 1× PLB (*see* **Note 23**).

2. Rock the plate slowly several times to ensure that the cells are completely covered.

3. Rock the culture plate at room temperature for 25 min at setting 3 (mid-high speed).

4. Transfer the cell lysate to a microcentrifuge tube (*see* **Note 24**).

5. Use an aliquot of each experimental lysate to analyze expression of overexpressed protein, E2F1 in this experiment (*see* **Note 25** and Fig. 4b).

3.4 Detection of Luciferase Enzymatic Activity

1. Dispense 20 μL of cells lysate, in triplicates, in a 96-well luminometer plate.

2. Prepare the luminometer with sufficient LAR II and Stop & Glo® reagents in order to dispense 100 μL per well.

3. Set the luminometer to first inject LAR II, read at 560 nm for 10 s (firefly luciferase), then inject Stop & Glo and read at 480 nm (*Renilla*) (*see* **Note 26**).

4. Obtain the readout and process the data in an excel spreadsheet (Table 2) (*see* **Note 27**).

5. Normalize data and represent in a graph (Table 1, Fig. 4a) (*see* **Note 28**).

---

4 Notes

1. The 293T cell line, originally referred as 293tsA1609neo, is a highly transfectable derivative of human embryonic kidney 293 cells, has epithelial morphology and grow adherent to the plastic surface.

2. Store it at 4 °C no longer than 4 weeks. Prewarm it in a water bath at 37 °C before use.

3. Before use, prewarm it at room temperature to ensure efficient detachment of adherent cells from the place surface.

Table 2
Example of a dual luciferase experiment set up

ng of vector	pRc-CMV-E2F1	pRL-TK *Renilla*	pGL3 3x-wtE2F	pGL3 3x-mutE2F	pRc-pCMV empty vector
3x-wtE2F LUC	0	20	200	0	1780
	100	20	200	0	1680
	200	20	200	0	1580
	500	20	200	0	1280
	1000	20	200	0	780
3x-mutE2F LUC	0	20	0	200	1780
	100	20	0	200	1680
	200	20	0	200	1580
	500	20	0	200	1280
	1000	20	0	200	780

Transfection mixes containing the plasmid DNA. 200 ng of target pGL3 plasmid (firefly) and 20 ng of pRL-TK control vector (Renilla) are added to all the mixes. Additionally, increasing amounts of pRc-CMV-E2F1 vector are added to the mixes. pRc-CMV empty vector is supplemented to have a total amount of 2 µg plasmid DNA in all the mixes

4. Caution should be used with Trypan Blue since it is a cancer suspect agent.

5. Wash both the Neubauer chamber and coverslip with %95 ethanol. Let ethanol evaporate before use. Mount the hemocytometer by placing the coverslip over the counting surface.

6. pRc-CMV-E2F1 is a mammalian expression plasmid that constitutively expresses human E2F1 and pRc-CMV is the empty vector control. pGL3 vectors express firefly luciferase regulated by the transcriptional potential of the sequence cloned upstream. All of them have been previously described [9, 13, 14].

7. X-tremeGENE HP DNA Transfection Reagent is a high-performance transfection reagent, free of animal-derived components. Benefits of X-tremeGENE HP DNA Transfection Reagent is that it is designed to transfect a broad range of eukaryotic cells, including insect cells, many cell lines not transfected well by other reagents, and hard-to-transfect cell lines (e.g., HT-1080, K-562, and HepG2). It produces minimal cytotoxicity or changes in morphology when adequate numbers of cells are transfected, eliminating the requirement to change media after adding the transfection complex. Store X-tremeGENE HP DNA Transfection Reagent at −15 to −25 °C, with the lid tightly closed. The reagent is stable until the expiration date printed on the label when stored under these conditions.

Special Handling of this reagent:

(a) After removing the amount required, tightly close the vial with the lid immediately after use.

(b) Always bring the vial to +15 to +25 °C and mix X-tremeGENE HP DNA Transfection Reagent prior to removing the amount required by vortexing for 1 s.

(c) Do not aliquot X-tremeGENE HP DNA Transfection Reagent; store in the original glass vials.

(d) Minimize the contact of undiluted X-tremeGENE HP DNA Transfection Reagent with plastic surfaces.

(e) For use, the minimum amount of X-tremeGENE HP DNA Transfection Reagent: DNA complex is 100 μL. Complex formation at lower volumes can significantly decrease transfection efficiency.

(f) Do not use tubes or microplates made of polystyrene for X-tremeGENE HP Transfection Reagent: DNA complex preparation. When not able to avoid polystyrene materials, make certain to pipet the transfection reagent directly into the serum-free medium (e.g., Opti-MEM).

(g) Do not use siliconized pipette tips or tubes.

8. Although serum-free DMEM media can also be used, Gibco™ Opti-MEM™ media is preferred as it contains additional supplements including insulin, transferrin, hypoxanthine, thymidine, and trace elements, which allow for a significant reduction in serum supplementation while maintaining cells in healthy conditions during transfection. Serum negatively affects transfection efficiency in a wide variety of cells. So it is recommended to use Opti-MEM when complex DNA and transfection reagents, such as X-tremeGENE HP DNA Transfection Reagent are employed. In addition, Opti-MEM is better buffered than DMEM, with a higher concentration of HEPES and sodium bicarbonate, which helps maintain cells healthy during transfection procedures.

9. PLB is specifically formulated to promote rapid lysis of cultured mammalian cells without the need to scrape adherent cells or perform additional freeze-thaw cycles (active lysis). Furthermore, PLB prevents sample foaming, making it ideally suited for high-throughput applications in which arrays of treated cells are cultured in multiwell plates, processed into lysates and assayed using automated systems.

10. Once reconstituted, the Luciferase Assay Substrate should be divided into aliquots and stored at −20 °C for up to 1 month or at −70 °C for up to 1 year.

11. First transfer 200 μL of Stop & Glo® Substrate Solvent into the amber glass vial containing dried Stop & Glo® Substrate and

mix well ("50×" stock solution). Then, add 1 volume of reconstituted 50× Stop & Glo® Substrate to 50 volumes of Stop Glo Buffer in a glass tube ("Stop & Glo® Reagent") (for example 50 μL of 50× Stop & Glo® Substrate + 2.5 mL of Stop & Glo® Buffer in glass tube). Ideally Stop & Glo® Reagent (Substrate + Buffer) should be freshly prepared before each use. If necessary, it can be stored at −20 °C for 15 days with no decrease in activity. If stored at 22 °C for 48 h, the reagent's activity decreases by 8%, and if stored at 4 °C for 15 days, the reagent's activity decreases by 13%. The Stop & Glo® Reagent can be thawed at room temperature up to 6 times with ≤15% decrease in activity.

12. The Clarity™ Luminescence Microplate Reader has been specifically designed for the detection of chemiluminescence and bioluminescence. It can be employed for all measurements of glow and flash luminescence in 96- or 384-well microplates. The luminometer utilizes high precision reagent injectors in combination with an ultrasensitive photon counting photomultiplier tube (PMT) detector, which are controlled using external PC software. Each injector uses microprocessor-controlled syringes to deliver exact amounts from 10 to 150 μL of reagent through chemically inert tubing to a disposable injector tip adjacent to the detector. Clarity supports the following protocol types: Raw Data, Fast Kinetics, Dual Measurement, and Batch Protocol. Users can create custom protocols for immediate use or store them for later availability. The Clarity protocol interface allows users to modify parameters such as injection volume, delay time, and measurement duration. The software easily formats to interchange 96- and 384-well microplates. Any combination of wells can be read. For detailed data analysis, Bio-Tek's KC4™ Data Analysis Software can be used. Single sample luminometers designed for low-throughput applications are also available. Promega™ Turner Designs TD-20/20 is one example, in which the reagents are added manually by pipetting and the reading is controlled by the user in the "LARII-Read-Stop&Glo®-read" format. For convenience, it is preferable to equip the luminometer with a printer for direct capture of data output, which eliminates having to stop after each measurement to manually record the measured values.

13. Make sure that culture media covers homogeneously the whole cell monolayer. Addition of at least 10 mL and 2 mL of media are recommended when using 10 cm culture dish and 6-well/plate, respectively.

14. Adherent cultures should be subcultured when they are in log phase, before they reach confluence. Normal cells stop growing when they reach confluence due to the contact inhibition

effect and it takes them longer to recover when reseeded. Transformed cells can proliferate even after they reach confluence, but they usually deteriorate after about two doublings. Hence, depending on the cell line used, splitting should be carried out every 2 or 3 days using 1:4–1:10 dilution so that the confluence does not exceed 90%.

15. Note that incubation time varies with the cell line used. Gently rock the plate to get complete coverage of the cell layer. Observe the cells under the microscope and if <90% of them are detached, increase the incubation time a few more minutes, checking for dissociation every 30 s.

16. Trypan Blue is a staining method also known as dye exclusion staining. It uses a diazo dye that selectively penetrates cell membranes of dead cells, coloring them blue, whereas it is not absorbed by membrane of viable cells, thus excluding living cells from staining.

17. Gently, expel the sample in the edge of the cover slip and allow the area underneath to fill by capillary action. Enough liquid should be introduced so that the mirrored surface is just covered, usually around 10 µL is sufficient. Be careful not to overfill the chambers since this will cause counting errors. Place the loaded hemocytometer on the microscope stage and count the live, unstained cells. Suspensions should be diluted enough so that the cells do not overlap each other on the grid, and should be uniformly distributed. The optimal number of cells to be counted is 1×10^5 cells/mL.

18. Gently move the place containing cell suspension to make sure cells are homogeneously distributed.

19. To help ensure independent genetic expression between experimental and control reporter genes it is recommended to perform preliminary cotransfection experiments to optimize both the amount of vector DNA and the ratio of coreporter vectors added to the transfection mix. Typically, 10:1–50:1 (or greater) for experimental vector–control reporter vector combinations are feasible and may aid greatly in suppressing the occurrence of trans effects between promoters.

20. Typically, dose-dependent effects of E2F1 expression might be considered, for example, by transfecting 0, 100, 200, 500, and 1000 ng of pRc-CMV-E2F1 expression vector. In order to keep constant the total amount of 2 µg of vectors in all the samples, the quantity of empty pRc-CMV vector to add in the tubes is 1780 ng, 1680 ng, 1580 ng, 1278 ng, and 780 ng, respectively.

21. Guidelines for preparing X-tremeGENE HP DNA Transfection Reagent: DNA Complex for Various Culture Vessel Sizes (http://www.sigmaaldrich.com/content/dam/sigma-aldrich/docs/Roche/Bulletin/1/xtghprobul.pdf). Also, it is

recommended to perform various sets of experiments and for that purpose it is recommended to prepare a master mix of transfection reagents for the total amount of replicates.

22. Cell confluence should be around 50–60% at the moment of transfection. Make sure that upon transfection cells proliferate efficiently, the color of the media must change (pH indicator).

23. Add a sufficient volume of 1× PLB to cover the cells (500 μL for each well of a 6-well plate).

24. The extracts may be assayed directly or stored at −70 °C.

25. This is a good control to correlate the relative expression of the transcription factor, E2F1 in this experiment, to the magnitude of luciferase activity. The antibody used in this control could be specific to E2F1. In this case, both endogenous and exogenous E2F1 would be detected. If the exogenous protein is tagged, for example with HA or FLAG, it can be detected specifically using anti-HA or anti-FLAG antibodies.

26. Follow carefully the users' guide provided with the luminometer. Before performing the experiment, make sure that the injectors are completely loaded with the reagents to use. And after obtaining the readout, proceed immediately to clean the injectors. Proper cleaning of an injector system exposed to Stop & Glo® Reagent is essential if the device is to be later used to perform firefly luciferase assays by autoinjecting LAR II. One of the luciferase-quenching components in Stop & Glo® Reagent has a moderate affinity for plastic materials. This compound exhibits a reversible association with the interior surfaces of plastic tubing and pump bodies commonly used in the construction of autoinjector systems.

27. Note that for each well there will be two readouts: one corresponding to the inducible firefly luciferase activity, and the other one corresponding to the constitutive *Renilla* luciferase activity.

28. A single experiment includes identical transfections in triplicate for each test group. Each sample is normalized by dividing the test reporter (Firefly luciferase) activity by the control reporter (*Renilla* luciferase) activity. Triplicate samples corresponding to the basal condition (with no pRc-CMV-E2F1 transfection) are averaged and given the relative luciferase unit (RLU) of 100. The normalized RLU % of control of the rest of the samples is calculated using the following equation:

$$ RLU \text{ \% control} = \frac{\left[(Firely / Renilla) \text{ from Sample A replica 1} \right] \times 100}{Average \text{ basal condition}} $$

Finally, triplicate samples are averaged and the standard deviation is calculated. This is done for each test group (Table 2).

Acknowledgments

This work was supported by grants from the Spanish Ministry (SAF2015-67562-R, cofunded by the European Regional Development fund) and the Basque Government (IT634-13 and KK-2015/89) to A.M.Z.

References

1. Manning AL, Dyson NJ (2011) pRB, a tumor suppressor with a stabilizing presence. Trends Cell Biol 21:433–441

2. Van Den Heuvel S, Dyson NJ (2008) Conserved functions of the pRB and E2F families. Nat Rev Mol Cell Biol 9:713–724

3. Ghim CM, Lee SK, Takayama S, Mitchell RJ (2010) The art of reporter proteins in science: past, present and future applications. BMB Rep 43(7):451–460

4. Zhu L, Zhu L, Xie E, Chang LS (1995) Differential roles of two tandem E2F sites in repression of the human p107 promoter by retinoblastoma and p107 proteins. Mol Cell Biol 15(7):3552–3562

5. Huang DY, Prystowsky MB (1996) Identification of an essential cis-element near the transcription start site for transcriptional activation of the proliferating cell nuclear antigen gene. J Biol Chem 271(2):1218–1225

6. Carrassa L, Broggini M, Vikhanskaya F, Damia G (2003) Characterization of the 5' flanking region of the human Chk1 gene: identification of E2F1 functional sites. Cell Cycle 2:604–609

7. Kherrouche Z, Blais A, Ferreira E, De Launoit Y, Monté D (2006) ASK-1 (apoptosis signal-regulating kinase 1) is a direct E2F target gene. Biochem J 396(3):547–556

8. Lu Z, Luo RZ, Peng H, Huang M, Nishmoto A, Hunt KK, Helin K, Liao WS, Yu Y (2006) E2F-HDAC complexes negatively regulate the tumor suppressor gene ARHI in breast cancer. Oncogene 25(2):230–239

9. Borah S, Verma SC, Robertson ES (2004) ORF73 of herpesvirus saimiri, a viral homolog of Kaposi's sarcoma-associated herpesvirus, modulates the two cellular tumor suppressor proteins p53 and pRb. J Virol 78: 10336–10347

10. Laresgoiti U, Apraiz A, Olea M, Mitxelena J, Osinalde N, Rodriguez JA, Fullaondo A, Zubiaga AM (2013) E2F2 and CREB cooperatively regulate transcriptional activity of cell cycle genes. Nucleic Acids Res 41(22): 10185–10198

11. Osinalde N, Olea M, Mitxelena J, Aloria K, Rodriguez JA, Fullaondo A, Arizmendi JM, Zubiaga AM (2013) The nuclear protein ALY binds to and modulates the activity of transcription factor E2F2. Mol Cell Proteomics 12(5): 1087–1098

12. Sherf BA, Navarro SL, Hannah RR, Wood V (1996) Dual-Luciferase® reporter assay: an advanced co-reporter technology integrating firefly and Renilla luciferase assays. Promega Notes 57:2–9

13. Krek W, Ewen ME, Shirodkar S, Arany Z, Kaelin WG Jr, Livingston DM (1994) Negative regulation of the growth promoting transcription factor E2F-1 by a stably bound cyclin A-dependent protein kinase. Cell 78:161–172

14. Krek W, Livingston DM, Shirodkar S (1993) Binding to DNA and the retinoblastoma gene product promoted by complex formation of different E2F family members. Science 262: 1557–1560

Chapter 15

Detection of HPV E6/E7 mRNA in Clinical Samples Using RNA In Situ Hybridization

Manishkumar Pandey, Priyanka G. Bhosale, and Manoj B. Mahimkar

Abstract

Detection of human papilloma virus (HPV) in tissue specimens has been a clinical challenge since last 2 decades; however, screening for presence of E6/E7 transcripts is regarded as the gold standard, and it verifies the active HPV infection. Here, we describe "RNAscope® assay" a novel RNA in situ hybridization (ISH) technology; which detects E6/E7 mRNA of seven high risk HPV subtypes (HPV 16, 18, 31, 33, 35, 52, and 58) in formalin fixed paraffin embedded (FFPE) tissue samples.

Key words HPV, E6/E7 mRNA, RNA in situ Hybridization, RNAscope®, HNSCC

1 Introduction

The role of high-risk human papilloma virus (HPV) in the development of subset of head and neck squamous cell carcinoma (HNSCC) has emphasized the need of a clinically apt algorithm for HPV detection [1, 2]. DNA in situ hybridization (DNA-ISH) and/or immunohistochemical (IHC) assays are commonly employed to screen for the presence of HPV DNA and protein biomarkers, respectively, in tissue samples [3, 4]. Detection of p16 INK4 A (p16) overexpression followed by screening of HPV DNA is a widely used method [5], however, presence of E6/E7 mRNA is regarded as the gold standard for the detection of transcriptionally active HPV infection, as it also substantiates role of HPV in malignant transformation of cells [6–8]. Real-time PCR is widely employed molecular technique to detect E6/E7 mRNA [9], however, this process involves laborious extraction procedures and it is impossible to map the observed signals to individual cells. Hence, it is challenging to develop a consensus approach for screening and detection of HPV in clinical samples with respect to sensitivity and specificity [10]. Here we demonstrate RNAscope®, a novel RNA in situ hybridization (RNA ISH) method that enables simultaneous detection of E6/E7 mRNA of seven high risk HPV subtypes (HPV 16, 18, 31, 33, 35, 52 and

Pedro G. Santiago-Cardona (ed.), *The Retinoblastoma Protein*, Methods in Molecular Biology, vol. 1726,
https://doi.org/10.1007/978-1-4939-7565-5_15, © Springer Science+Business Media, LLC 2018

58) in formalin fixed paraffin embedded (FFPE) tissues. RNAscope®, a product of Advance Cell Diagnostics (Hayward, CA, USA), is an explicit and sensitive method that utilizes oligonucleotide probes for seven high-risk HPV, an internal positive control probe for Ubiquitin C gene and internal negative control for bacterial gene dapB. Additionally, unique probe design strategy with signal amplification system allows single molecule visualization in individual cells and makes this assay a promising technique for HPV detection in clinical specimens [11–14].

2   Materials

This chapter details detection of HPV (RNAscope® Probe-HPV-HR7 Cat No. 312351) in FFPE tissues using RNAscope® 2.5 HD Reagent Kit-Brown. Prepare all the reagents in Milli-Q® water (prepared by purifying deionized water, to attain a sensitivity of 18 MΩ/cm at 25 °C) and store at indicated temperatures. Perform all the incubations at specified temperatures. Set Hybridization Oven/Incubator at 40 °C at least 30 min before starting the procedure. Place a humidifying paper in the humidity control tray and wet completely with distilled water (*see* **Note 1**). Warm the tray to 40 °C at least 30 min before use.

2.1 Tissue Processing and Pretreatment

1. Xylene.
2. 100%, 95%, 70% ethanol (EtOH).
3. 0.5% Harris Hematoxylin solution.
4. DPX mountant.
5. Poly-L-lysine coated slides.

2.2 RNAscope Reagent Preparation

1. 1× Pretreat 2 (RNAscope® Target Retrieval Reagent provided with the kit): Prepare 700 mL of RNAscope® 1× Target Retrieval Reagent just before use by adding 630 mL distilled water to 70 mL, 10× Target Retrieval Reagent. Mix well (*see* **Note 2**).

2. 1× Wash Buffer: Warm RNAscope® 50× Wash Buffer (provided with the kit) at 40 °C for 10–20 min before preparation. Prepare 3 L of 1× Wash Buffer in a large carboy by adding 2.94 L distilled water and 1 bottle (60 mL) of RNAscope® Wash Buffer (50×). Mix well and store at room temperature (RT) for up to 1 month.

3. Reagent Equilibration: Before each use equilibrate AMP 1–6 reagents (provided with the kit) for at least 30 min at room temperature and warm the Target as well as Control probes for at least 10 min in a water bath or incubator set at 40 °C.

4. 24 mm × 60 mm coverslips.

3 Methods

3.1 Pretreatment of FFPE Tissue Sample

1. Three FFPE tissue sections per tissue (For HPV, UBC, and DapB probe treatment) present on poly-L-lysine coated slides are to be processed as described below.

2. Bake slides in a dry oven for 1 h at 60 °C (Optional stopping point: use immediately or store slides for ≥1 week at RT with desiccants). *See* **Note 3**.

3. Incubate the slides in xylene for 5 min at RT. Agitate the slides by occasionally lifting the slide rack up and down in the dish.

4. Remove the slide rack from the first xylene-containing dish and immediately place in the second xylene-containing dish at RT for 5 min.

5. Remove the slide rack from the second xylene-containing dish and immediately place in the dish containing 100% EtOH.

6. Incubate the slides in 100% EtOH for 1 min at RT with slight agitation.

7. Repeat **steps 5** and **6** with fresh 100% EtOH.

8. Remove the slides from the rack, and place on absorbent paper with the section face-up. Air-dry slides for 5 min at RT (or until completely dry).

3.2 Pretreatment 1: Hydrogen Peroxide Blocking

1. Add 5–8 drops of RNAscope® Hydrogen Peroxide (provided with the kit) to each section and incubate for 10 min at RT.

2. Remove hydrogen peroxide solution from one slide at a time by tapping and/or flicking the slide on absorbent paper.

3. Wash the slide in distilled water by moving the slide rack up and down 3–5 times and repeat with fresh distilled water.

3.3 Pretreatment 2: RNAscope® Target Retrieval

1. Place the beaker containing 200 mL RNAscope® 1× Target Retrieval Reagent (provided with the kit) on the hot plate. Cover the beaker with foil and turn the hot plate on high for 10–15 min.

2. Once 1× RNAscope® Target Retrieval Reagent starts boiling, turn the hot plate to a lower setting to maintain the temperature of around (98–102 °C). Check the temperature with a thermometer (*see* **Note 4**).

3. Transfer slides to boiling 1× target retrieval solution (98–102 °C) and incubate for 15 min (*see* **Note 5**).

4. Immediately transfer the slides into the beaker/Coplin jar containing distilled water at RT.

5. Wash the slides in fresh distilled water by moving the slides up and down 3–5 times, repeat with fresh distilled water.

6. Transfer the slides to fresh 100% EtOH and wash by moving the rack up and down 3–5 times. Air-dry the slides (*see* **Note 6**).

**3.4 Creating
a Hydrophobic Barrier**

1. Using a hydrophobic barrier pen provided with the kit (Immedge) or using alternatives create a hydrophobic barrier around each section (Fig. 1) so that the solution/reagent will not overflow the tissue or will be in close proximity of the tissue (*see* **Note 7**).

2. Dry completely for 2 min or overnight at RT (Optional stopping point: Dry slides at RT for overnight, must be used within 24 h or proceed directly to the next step).

**3.5 Pretreatment 3:
Protease Treatment**

1. Add 5–6 drops of Pretreat 3 solutions (protease provided with the kit) to entirely cover the sections.

2. Place the slides in a humidity control tray and incubate for 30 min at 40 °C. Prepare RNAscope® 2.5 Assay Reagent (*see* **Note 8**).

3. Wash the slides in distilled water by moving the slide rack up and down 3–5 times and repeat with fresh distilled water.

**3.6 RNAscope®
2.5 Assay**

3.6.1 Probe Hybridization

1. Tap to remove excess liquid from slides and place in the humidified control tray. Add ~4 drops of the appropriate probe (provided with the kit) to entirely cover each section (Fig. 1).

2. Cover the humidity control tray with lid and insert into the oven for 2 h at 40 °C.

3. Remove excess liquid by tapping the slide on humidifying or blotting paper, place the slide in slide rack and submerged the slide rack in dish containing 1× Wash Buffer.

4. Wash the slides in 1× Wash Buffer for 2 min at RT. Move the slide rack up and down in between.

*3.6.2 AMP 1
Hybridization*

1. Tap to remove excess liquid from slides and place in the humidified control tray. Add 4–5 drops of AMP 1 (provided with the kit) to entirely cover each section.

2. Close tray and insert into the oven for 30 min at 40 °C.

3. Remove excess liquid by tapping the slide on humidifying or blotting paper, place the slide in slide rack and submerge the slide rack in dish containing 1× Wash Buffer.

4. Wash slides in 1× Wash Buffer for 2 min at RT with occasional agitation.

5. Repeat **step 4** with fresh 1× Wash Buffer.

*3.6.3 AMP 2
Hybridization*

1. Tap to remove excess liquid from slides and place in the humidified control tray. Add 4–5 drops of AMP 2 (provided with the kit) to entirely cover each section.

2. Close tray and insert into the oven for 15 min at 40 °C.

3. Remove excess liquid by tapping the slide on humidifying or blotting paper, place the slide in slide rack and submerge the slide rack in dish containing 1× Wash Buffer.

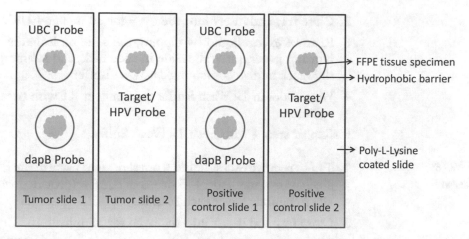

UBC Probe

UBC Probe

Target/
HPV Probe

Target/
HPV Probe → FFPE tissue specimen
→ Hydrophobic barrier

dapB Probe

dapB Probe

→ Poly-L-Lysine
coated slide

Tumor slide 1   Tumor slide 2   Positive
control slide 1   Positive
control slide 2

Fig. 1 Diagrammatic representation of tissue section arrangement for RNAscope® assay

4. Wash slides in 1× Wash Buffer for 2 min at RT with occasional agitation.

5. Repeat **step 4** with fresh 1× Wash Buffer.

3.6.4 AMP 3
Hybridization

1. Tap to remove excess liquid from slides and place in the humidified control tray. Add 4–5 drops of AMP 3 (provided with the kit) to entirely cover each section.

2. Close tray and insert into the oven for 30 min at 40 °C.

3. Remove excess liquid by tapping the slide on humidifying or blotting paper, place the slide in slide rack and submerge the slide rack in dish containing 1× Wash Buffer.

4. Wash slides in 1× Wash Buffer for 2 min at RT with occasional agitation.

5. Repeat **step 4** with fresh 1× Wash Buffer.

3.6.5 AMP 4
Hybridization

1. Tap to remove excess liquid from slides and place in the humidified control tray. Add 4–5 drops of AMP 4 (provided with the kit) to entirely cover each section.

2. Close tray and insert into the oven for 15 min at 40 °C.

3. Remove excess liquid by tapping the slide on humidifying or blotting paper, place the slide in slide rack and submerge the slide rack in dish containing 1× Wash Buffer.

4. Wash slides in 1× Wash Buffer for 2 min at RT with occasional agitation.

5. Repeat **step 4** with fresh 1× Wash Buffer.

3.6.6 AMP 5
Hybridization

1. Tap to remove excess liquid from slides and place in the humidified control tray. Add 4–5 drops of AMP 5 (provided with the kit) to entirely cover each section (*see* **Note 9**).

2. Close tray and insert into the oven for 30 min at 40 °C.

3. Remove excess liquid by tapping the slide on humidifying or blotting paper, place the slide in slide rack, and submerge the slide rack in dish containing 1× Wash Buffer.

4. Wash slides in 1× Wash Buffer for 2 min at RT with occasional agitation.

5. Repeat **step 4** with fresh 1× Wash Buffer.

3.6.7 AMP 6
Hybridization

1. Tap to remove excess liquid from slides and place in the humidified control tray. Add 4–5 drops of AMP 6 (provided with the kit) to entirely cover each section.

2. Close tray and insert into the oven for 15 min at 40 °C.

3. Remove excess liquid by tapping the slide on humidifying or blotting paper, place the slide in slide rack and submerge the slide rack in dish containing 1× Wash Buffer.

4. Wash slides in 1× Wash Buffer for 2 min at RT with occasional agitation.

5. Repeat **step 4** with fresh 1× Wash Buffer.

3.6.8 Signal Detection

1. Mix equal volumes of DAB-A and DAB-B (provided with kit) in an appropriately sized tube by dispensing the same number of drops of each solution. Make DAB substrate depending on tissue size; ~120 μL per section (~2 drops of each reagent). Mix well 3–5 times.

2. Remove excess liquid by tapping the slide on humidifying or blotting paper.

3. Pipette ~120 μL of DAB onto each tissue section. Ensure sections are covered, and incubate for 10 min at RT.

4. Insert the slide into a slide rack submerged in a staining dish filled with tap water.

3.6.9 Counterstaining

1. Immerse the slide rack in dish containing 0.5% Harris Hematoxylin solution (not provided with the kit) and incubate for 2 min at RT.

2. Immediately transfer the slide rack back into the staining dish containing tap water, and wash slides 3–5 times by moving the rack up and down. Keep repeating with fresh tap water until the slides are clear, while sections remain purple.

3.6.10 Dehydration

1. Transfer the slide rack in a dish containing 70% EtOH for 2 min with occasional agitation.

2. Transfer the slide rack in a dish containing 95% EtOH for 2 min with occasional agitation.

3. Transfer the slide rack in a new dish containing 95% EtOH for 2 min with occasional agitation.

4. Transfer the slide rack in dish containing xylene for 5 min with occasional agitation.

5. Air-dry the slide for 5 min at RT or until completely dry.

3.6.11 Mounting

1. Remove the slides from the slide rack and lay flat with the sections facing up.

2. Mount one slide at a time by adding 1 drop of DPX mountant (xylene-based mounting medium) to each slide and carefully placing a 24 mm × 60 mm coverslip over the section. Avoid trapping air bubbles.

3. Incubate the slides at 37 °C for 5 min or till the mountant is completely dry.

3.6.12 Sample Evaluation Guidelines

1. The RNAscope® Assay enhances the value of in situ hybridization results by enabling a semiquantitative scoring guideline utilizing the estimated number of punctate dots present within each cell boundary.

2. Guidelines for semiquantitative assessment of RNAscope® staining intensity is presented in Table 1 for HPV E6/E7 gene expression level varying between 1 to >10 copies per cell. The scale criteria can be modified accordingly for a gene with expression level higher or lower than this range.

3. For each HNSCC case, all 3 stained sections/slides (HPV, UBC, and dapB) were examined simultaneously by the pathologist to determine the HPV status (*see* **Note 10**). The UBC test was used to assess the presence of hybridizable RNA; if the UBC slide was negative, the sample was disqualified, presuming insufficient RNA quality. The dapB test was used to assess nonspecific staining; only those cases that were negative or had weak staining were considered for HPV scoring (*see* **Note 11**). A positive HPV test result was defined as punctate staining that colocalized to the cytoplasm or nucleus of the malignant cells (Fig. 2).

4 Notes

1. Incubation steps in the RNAscope® assay require humid condition to prevent sections from drying out.

2. Prepare 1× Pretreat 2 reagent (RNAscope® Target Retrieval Reagent) before 30 min. Do not store for later use, and hence prepare as per requirement.

Table 1
RNAscope® staining intensity scoring criteria

Staining score	Microscope objective scoring
0	No staining or <1 dot to every 10 cells (40× magnification)
1	1–3 dots/cell (visible at 20–40× magnification)
2	4–10 dots/cell. Very few dot clusters (visible at 20–40× magnification)
3	>10 dots/cell. Less than 10% positive cells have dot clusters (visible at 20× magnification)
4	>10 dots/cell. More than 10% positive cells have dot clusters (visible at 20× magnification)

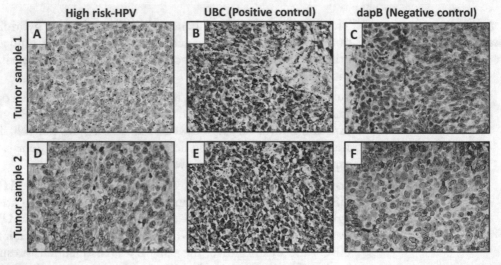

Fig. 2 Detection of high-risk human papilloma virus (HPV) RNA in HNSCC tumor samples. RNA in situ hybridization (ISH) showing punctate brown signals for HR-HPV RNA in tumor sample 1 (**a**), and its respective internal positive control (**b**). HPV negative tumor sample 2 with no signal for HR-HPV RNA (**d**), and punctate brown signals for internal positive control (**e**). No signals were observed in internal negative controls (**c, f**) in either case

3. Slides baked in dry oven for 1 h at 60 °C must be used immediately or within a week as prolonged storage of baked slide may degrade the RNA quality.

4. Do not boil 1× RNAscope® target retrieval buffer for more than 30 min.

5. Tissue sections on slide must be submerged in RNAscope® target retrieval buffer during the target retrieval process, failing to which may result in nonspecific signals.

6. Do not let your sections dry out during the procedure (except wherever specified).

7. While drawing the hydrophobic barrier around the tissue section, do not allow the hydrophobic barrier to touch the tissue section.

8. Equilibrate AMP 1–6 reagents (provided with the kit) for at least 30 min at room temperature and warm the Target as well as Control probes for at least 10 min in a water bath or incubator set at 40 °C.

9. Staining intensity can be modified by adjusting the AMP 5 incubation time.

10. For data interpretation evaluate the slides from two independent pathologists.

11. Always run positive and negative control probes on your sample to assess sample RNA quality and optimal assay workflow for result interpretation. Also run a positive control sample with each batch to assess batch variation (Fig. 1).

References

1. Adamopoulou M et al (2013) Prevalence of human papillomavirus in saliva and cervix of sexually active women. Gynecol Oncol 129(2):395–400

2. Braakhuis BJ et al (2009) Human papilloma virus in head and neck cancer: the need for a standardised assay to assess the full clinical importance. Eur J Cancer 45(17):2935–2939

3. Levsky JM, Singer RH (2003) Fluorescence in situ hybridization: past, present and future. J Cell Sci 116(Pt 14):2833–2838

4. Matos LL et al (2010) Immunohistochemistry as an important tool in biomarkers detection and clinical practice. Biomark Insights 5:9–20

5. Hoffmann M et al (2012) HPV DNA, E6*I-mRNA expression and p16INK4A immunohistochemistry in head and neck cancer - how valid is p16INK4A as surrogate marker? Cancer Lett 323(1):88–96

6. Mirghani H et al (2014) Human papilloma virus testing in oropharyngeal squamous cell carcinoma: what the clinician should know. Oral Oncol 50(1):1–9

7. van Houten VM et al (2001) Biological evidence that human papillomaviruses are etiologically involved in a subgroup of head and neck squamous cell carcinomas. Int J Cancer 93(2):232–235

8. Jung AC et al (2010) Biological and clinical relevance of transcriptionally active human papillomavirus (HPV) infection in oropharynx squamous cell carcinoma. Int J Cancer 126(8):1882–1894

9. Sotiriou C, Piccart MJ (2007) Taking gene-expression profiling to the clinic: when will molecular signatures become relevant to patient care? Nat Rev Cancer 7(7):545–553

10. Bhosale PG et al (2016) Low prevalence of transcriptionally active human papilloma virus in Indian patients with HNSCC and leukoplakia. Oral Surg Oral Med Oral Pathol Oral Radiol 122(5):609–618e7

11. Wang F et al (2012) RNAscope: a novel in situ RNA analysis platform for formalin-fixed, paraffin-embedded tissues. J Mol Diagn 14(1):22–29

12. Bishop JA et al (2012) Detection of transcriptionally active high-risk HPV in patients with head and neck squamous cell carcinoma as visualized by a novel E6/E7 mRNA in situ hybridization method. Am J Surg Pathol 36(12):1874–1882

13. Ukpo OC et al (2011) High-risk human papillomavirus E6/E7 mRNA detection by a novel in situ hybridization assay strongly correlates with p16 expression and patient outcomes in oropharyngeal squamous cell carcinoma. Am J Surg Pathol 35(9):1343–1350

14. Wang H et al (2014) RNAscope for in situ detection of transcriptionally active human papillomavirus in head and neck squamous cell carcinoma. J Vis Exp 85

Chapter 16

CRISPR/Cas9-Mediated Knockout of *Rb1* in *Xenopus tropicalis*

Thomas Naert and Kris Vleminckx

Abstract

At this time, no molecular targeted therapies exist for treatment of retinoblastoma. This can be, in part, attributed to the lack of animal models that allow for both rapid identification of novel therapeutic targets and hypothesis driven drug testing. Within this scope, we have recently reported the first genuine genetic nonmammalian retinoblastoma cancer model within the aquatic model organism *Xenopus tropicalis* (Naert et al., Sci Rep 6: 35263, 2016). Here we describe the methods to generate *rb1* mosaic mutant *Xenopus tropicalis* by employing the CRISPR/Cas9 technology. In depth, we discuss short guide RNA (sgRNA) design parameters, generation, quality control, quantification, and delivery followed by several methods for assessing genome editing efficiencies. As such the reader should be capable, by minor changes to the methods described here, to (co-) target *rb1* or any one or multiple gene(s) within the *Xenopus tropicalis* genome by multiplex CRISPR/Cas9 methodology.

Key words *Xenopus tropicalis*, Disease model, Cancer model, Tumor model, Retinoblastoma, Genome editing, CRISPR/Cas9, Rb1

1 Introduction

Biallelic inactivation of *Retinoblastoma 1 (RB1)* is the initiating genetic lesion for development of retinoblastoma (OMIM: 180200), a pediatric cancer of the eye [1]. The study of the *RB1* gene was historically quintessential in delineating the concept of the two-hit model for tumor suppressor genes [2–4]. The model explained heritable, and usually bilateral, occurrence of retinoblastoma being due to the presence of a germ line mutation in one *RB1* allele followed by a somatic mutation in the other. Next to this, it provided an explanation for sporadic, and usually unilateral, retinoblastoma resulting from two independent somatic *RB1* mutations. Of note, *RB1* mutations are also associated with development of so-called trilateral retinoblastoma, a pediatric intracranial neuroblastic tumor, osteosarcomas, small cell lung cancer, and soft tissue cancers [5–10]. Considering that the existing retinoblastoma mice

Pedro G. Santiago-Cardona (ed.), *The Retinoblastoma Protein*, Methods in Molecular Biology, vol. 1726,
https://doi.org/10.1007/978-1-4939-7565-5_16, © Springer Science+Business Media, LLC 2018

models have already shown to be extremely valuable for preclinical research, we aimed to generate a novel, rapid, and highly penetrant nonmammalian model for retinoblastoma in the aquatic model organism *Xenopus tropicalis* [11–14]. The recent advances in genome engineering by targeted nucleases, most prominent by the CRISPR/Cas9 methodology, have enabled researchers to perform targeted genome editing in model organisms previously recalcitrant to genomic engineering, such as *Xenopus tropicalis (X. tropicalis)* [15]. Gene studies in these model organisms were historically limited to transient gene knockdown or large-scale random mutagenesis approaches [16]. However, with TALENs and CRISPR/Cas9 it is now possible to specifically target a gene of interest in these model organisms [17–19]. By employing the CRISPR/Cas9 system we have recently shown that CRISPR/Cas9-mediated knockout of *rb1* and *rbl1* leads to rapid and penetrant retinoblastoma development in *X. tropicalis* [20]. In our opinion, the described methods for CRISPR/Cas9 mediated genome editing of members of the retinoblastoma protein family described in this chapter are applicable to any model organism where the possibility exists to efficiently deliver short guide RNA (sgRNA) and Cas9 protein to the early developing embryo. We demonstrate the possibility, and ease of use, for multiplex targeting of multiple genes and how this can overcome functional redundancy (*rb1* and *rbl1*). We speculate multiplex CRISPR/Cas9 to be applicable for overcoming redundancy in model organism with (pseudo) tetraploid genomes such as zebrafish. This chapter in length describes the process from in silico sgRNA design up to genotyping of the genome-edited F0 mosaic mutant animal. Additionally, small adaptions of this protocol should render the reader capable of efficiently targeting other tumor suppressors, or in fact any gene, by CRISPR/Cas9 technology in *Xenopus tropicalis*.

2   Materials

2.1 Generation of sgRNA DNA Template by the PCR Method

1. 5′ primer with the sequence: 'GAAT("oligo_from_CRISPRScan")ATAGC'. *See* Subheading 3.1 for explanation of target site choice.

2. 3′ primer with the sequence: 'AAAAGCACCGACTCGGTGCCACTTTTTCAAGTTGATAACGGACTAGCCTTATTTTAACTTGCTATTTCTAGCTCTAAAAC'

3. High-fidelity proof-reading polymerase (e.g., Velocity DNA polymerase, Bioline, BIO-21099). *See* **Note 1**.

4. 10 mM dNTP mix.

5. RNase-free water.

6. PureLink® PCR Purification Kit (ThermoFisher Scientific; K310001, *see* **Note 2**).

7. A NanoDrop instrument (ThermoFisher Scientific).

8. 1 kb DNA Ladder.

9. Thermocycler.

2.2 In Vitro Transcription of sgRNA

1. T7 MegaShortScript (ThermoFisher Scientific; AM1354), or HiScribe™ T7 High Yield RNA Synthesis Kit (NEB; E2040S). *See* **Note 3**.

2. TURBO™ DNase (ThermoFisher Scientific; AM2238). *See* **Note 4**.

3. Phenol–chloroform–isoamyl alcohol, 25:24:1.

4. Chloroform.

5. 5 M Ammonium Acetate. We buy this as a premade solution (e.g., ThermoFisher Scientific, AM9070G).

6. 100% EtOH (RNase-free).

2.3 Determination of sgRNA Quality by Denaturing Gel Electrophoresis

All glassware employed should be baked at 180 °C for 2 h to remove any RNase activity.

1. Diethyl pyrocarbonate (DEPC).

2. DEPC treated (RNase-free) water. Add 1% (w/v) DEPC to purified water and let incubate at room temperature under the fume hood. Make sure to thoroughly mix the DEPC every 2 h by shaking the bottle. This shaking needs to be done at least three times and should be followed by an overnight incubation. The DEPC-treated water is then autoclaved to degrade the DEPC.

3. 10× 3-(N-morpholino)propanesulfonic acid (MOPS) buffer: 20 mM EDTA, 200 mM MOPS, 50 mM sodium acetate, pH 7.0. Make this 10× stock with purified water. After setting correct pH by NaOH, add 1% DEPC and perform the same steps as described above for correct DEPC treatment of water. The 10× MOPS must then be autoclaved to break down the DEPC. The solution will turn straw-yellow and should be kept in the dark to prevent degradation. By this preparation method you inactivate any RNase present in your solid powder reagents used to prepare this buffer.

4. 37% formaldehyde.

5. RNA loading buffer. To prepare, dilute GelRed 10,000× (Biotium; #41003) to 1× working concentration in NorthernMax® Formaldehyde Load Dye (ThermoFisher Scientific; AM8552). *See* **Note 5**.

6. Quantitative RNA ladder (e.g., RiboRuler High Range RNA Ladder, ThermoFisher Scientific; SM1821).

7. Agarose kept under RNase-free conditions.

8. RNase Surface Decontaminant.

9. Gel Doc™ XR+ Gel Documentation System (Bio-Rad; **1708195**).

2.4 sgRNA Quantification

1. Image Lab™ Software 5.2.1 (Bio-Rad).

2. A Qubit™ fluorometer (e.g., Qubit™ 3.0 Fluorometer; ThermoFisher Scientific; Q33216).

3. Qubit® RNA BR Assay Kit (ThermoFisher Scientific; Q10210).

2.5 Delivery of sgRNA/Cas9 Ribonucleoproteins by Microinjection to Xenopus tropicalis Embryos

1. General microinjection equipment consisting of a stereomicroscope supplied with an ocular micrometer for calibration of the injection volume, a cold-light source, a 3D micromanipulator, and a microinjector.

2. Microinjection needles produced from borosilicate glass capillaries (with 1.0 and 0.58 mm as outer and inner diameter, respectively, using a micropipette puller.

3. Injection dish: a 60 mm petri dish in which a mesh (e.g., 700 μM mesh) is fixed with a few drops of chloroform.

4. Adult *Xenopus tropicalis* males and females.

5. Human chorionic gonadotropin (HCG).

6. 10× Marc's Modified Ringers (MMR) Solution: 1 M NaCl, 18 mM KCl, 20 mM $CaCl_2$, 10 mM $MgCl_2$, 50 mM Hepes, pH 7.6.

7. 6% (w/v) Ficoll 400 in 0.1× MMR.

8. 2% (w/v) cysteine solution in 0.1× MMR, adjusted to pH 8.0 with NaOH.

9. Commercially available recombinant injection-ready Cas9 protein (e.g., Toolgen Cas9 WT protein; TGEN_CP) or homemade NLS-Cas9-NLS can be prepared as described in supplementary materials of Naert et al. [20].

2.6 Assessment of Genome Editing in F0 Mosaic Mutant X. tropicalis

1. Lysis buffer: 50 mM Tris-HCl pH 8.8, 1 mM EDTA, 0.5% Tween 20, 200 μg/mL Proteinase K.

2. High-fidelity proof-reading polymerase (e.g., Phusion polymerase, ThermoFisher Scientific; F530).

3. 5× Tris-Borate-EDTA (TBE): 45 mM Tris-borate, 1 mM EDTA, pH 8.3.

4. Polyacrylamide gel electrophoresis system.

5. 10% Ammonium persulfate (APS) solution, we buy a premade solution (e.g., Sigma-Aldrich A3678).

6. Tetramethylethylenediamine (TEMED).

7. Acrylamide–Bis-acrylamide, 37.5:1, 40%.

8. DNA Gel Loading Dye.

9. GelRed 10,000× in water (Biotium; #41003) (*see* **Note 5**).

3   Methods

3.1   Design of sgRNAs

As the CRISPR/Cas9 technology became an established technique over the past few years, an ever increasing number of sgRNA design tools became available. Over the past years, we successfully employed different tools such as CCTOP, CRISPRDesign and CRISPRScan [21–23]. Currently, however, we are consistently using the CRISPRScan design tool which provides an in silico prediction of CRISPR/Cas9 modification efficiencies at the target sites and the employed algorithm is validated in *Xenopus tropicalis*. We have had a more than acceptable success rate with this tool and we would thus recommend it, at the time this chapter was written and in our hands, as the most efficient for design of sgRNA that will be delivered to embryos as purified RNA together with Cas9 protein.

As the goal in most of our set ups is to obtain a (tumor development) phenotype in F0 mosaic *X. tropicalis* animals, it is extremely important during the design phase, to not only attempt to maximize on-target sgRNA editing efficiency by employing predictive in silico design tools but also to target functional protein domains [23]. From the two-hit hypothesis, it becomes clear that both alleles of *rb1* (and potentially, depending on your specific needs and model organism of interest, *rbl1* and/or *rbl2*) need to be targeted by the CRISPR/Cas9 system in such a way that each allele leads to loss-of-function (LOF). Theoretically, one-third of the small insertion/deletions (indels) generated by the CRISPR/Cas9 system will be in frame and thus might not necessarily lead to LOF by non-sense mediated decay [24]. This phenomenon can strongly impact the possibility of phenotype development due to reduced number of cells containing no functional protein for this specific targeted gene.

The following steps outline how to design a highly active sgRNA targeting the E2F binding pocket of *rb1*. If you however choose to target another region of the *rb1* gene, keep in mind not to target the final exon of the gene or you will obtain 3′ truncated protein due to absence of nonsense-mediated decay of the transcript. Additionally, beware of targeting the first exon as editing there might give rise to 5′ truncated protein due to alternative start codon usage or alternative first exon usage.

1. Identify for the model organism of interest the genetic sequence coding the E2F binding pocket of your protein from the retinoblastoma family [25].

2. Browse the URL of the CRISPRScan design tool (http://www.crisprscan.org/; URL and website layout subject to change).

3. Choose the "Submit Sequence" tool at top left and input your target sequence as raw or FASTA data. Subsequently, choose your appropriate genomic off-target calculator to the right, in our case *Xenopus tropicalis*.

4. Click "get sgRNA" and subsequently immediately export your data by "options" → "export" → "tab-delimited".

5. The obtained sheet can be opened in excel and can be sorted (from high to low) according to CRISPRScan scores, which is a score assigned to the sgRNA based on the predictive algorithm of CRISPRScan. For more information on how these scores relate to in vivo effectiveness in our hands *see* **Note 6**.

6. Choose the highest scoring sgRNA. For this sgRNA keep handy the "oligo" output.

3.2 Generation of Microinjection-Ready sgRNA

Generation of sgRNAs is performed by a cloning-free method shown schematically in Fig. 1a [15]. Keep in mind that the first two nucleotides transcribed by the T7 RNA polymerase should be GG (*see* **Note 7**). Next to this we demonstrate methods for quality control of sgRNA and the best practice for quantification. During all steps of this protocol we recommend working as RNase free as possible, this includes using only RNase-free reagents, consumables, glassware, etc., while working in an environment thoroughly cleaned by RNase surface decontaminant and keeping any employed kits RNase free.

3.2.1 Generation of sgRNA DNA Templates by PCR Method

In order to obtain a linear DNA template for in vitro transcription of microinjection-ready sgRNA, we employ a PCR-based strategy to anneal a variable forward 5′ primer (modified according to the desired sgRNA target site) and a common 3′ primer.

1. Obtain the following oligos:

   Variable forward sgRNA targeting sequence containing 5′ primer: GAAT("oligo_from_CRISPRScan")ATAGC

   Constant reverse 3′ primer: AAAAGCACCGACTCGGT GCCACTTTTTCAAGTTGATAACGGACTAGCCTTAT TTTAACTTGCTATTTCTAGCTCTAAAAC

2. Set up the following DNA template generation reaction in a thermocycler (*see* **Note 1** on polymerase use). Please mind that 5′ and 3′ primers are added to this reaction at a 100 μM concentration.

   DNA template assembly reaction:

5× Hi-Fi Reaction buffer	10 μL
10 mM dNTP mix	5 μL
5′ primer (100 μM)	2 μL
3′ primer (100 μM)	2 μL
Velocity Hi-Fi Polymerase	1 μL
Purified water	30 μL

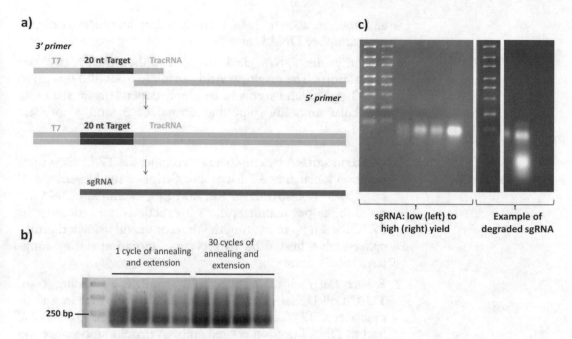

Fig. 1 Generation of sgRNA DNA templates by PCR method. (**a**) A variable 3′ primer specific to the sgRNA target site and a common 5′ primer are annealed and amplified in a PCR reaction generating large amounts of DNA template. This template will subsequently be used to generate sgRNA by in vitro transcription from the T7 promotor (grey). (**b**) Representative gel showing clear amplification of the correct DNA template fragment (~121 bp) when comparing 1 cycle of annealing and extension to 30 cycles of annealing and extension. (**c**) Representative denaturing RNA gel (left) showing two dilutions of the quantitative ladder with four sgRNAs exhibiting low to high sgRNA yield after in vitro transcription. Representative denaturing RNA gel (right; cut and pasted but ladder and sample are from the same gel) exhibiting sgRNA that has undergone degradation due to inappropriate sample handling. The employed ladder for both gels is the RiboRuler High Range RNA Ladder (ThermoFisher Scientific)

Run PCR reaction in a thermocycler with the following program: 98 °C for 2 min; 30 cycles of (98 °C for 30 s; 60 °C for 30 s; 72 °C for 15 s); 72 °C for 4 min. Correct amplification of the DNA template can be demonstrated by loading a control sample that only underwent one cycle of annealing and extension (program: 98 °C for 2 min; 1 cycle of [98 °C for 30 s; 60 °C for 30 s; 72 °C for 15 s]; 72 °C for 4 min).

3. Use 2 µL (1/25 of the total volume) to perform a quality control by gel electrophoresis with an appropriate DNA ladder. The obtained band should be 121 base pairs in size. and if including the negative control, this band should be more intense, thus demonstrating correct amplification. A representative gel is shown in Fig. 1b.

4. Cleanup the DNA template by PureLink® PCR Purification Kit or other equivalent column purification method. Mind to elute the template in RNase-free water and not the buffer suggested in the kit. Traditional phenol–chloroform extraction

and sodium acetate EtOH precipitation in order to obtain pure template DNA is also possible.

5. Quantify the DNA yield by spectrophotometry (we use NanoDrop). The resulting yield can range from 200 ng/μL to over 1 μg/μL and seems to be highly dependent on the exact molecular amounts (pipetting errors) of 5′ and 3′ primers added.

3.2.2 In Vitro Transcription of sgRNA

1. Generate sgRNA by employing a commercial T7 in vitro transcription kit such as T7 MegaShortScript or the HiScribe™T7 High Yield RNA Synthesis Kit. Add 1 μg of template DNA per reaction, as per manufacturer's instructions, and incubate at 37 °C for 4 h up to overnight. We recommend using a thermocycler with a heated lid to prevent evaporation during long-term incubations.

2. Ensure full removal of the DNA template by adding 1 μL TURBO™ DNase- treatment and incubate further in a thermocycler at 37 °C for 15 min (*see* **Note 4**). Failure to do so will lead to DNA injection related embryo toxicity upon injection of the sgRNAs.

3. Purify the sgRNAs by phenol–chloroform extraction (phenol–chloroform–isoamyl alcohol 25:24:1) and NH_4OAc/EtOH precipitation. Resuspend the pellet in 20 μL of DEPC-treated water.

3.2.3 sgRNA Quality Control by Denaturing Gel Electrophoresis

The generated sgRNA needs be quality controlled by running denaturing MOPS gel electrophoresis. This is necessary to verify that no degradation of the sgRNA took place during purification and for visual estimation of in vitro transcription yield by comparison with a quantitative RNA marker. Due to the formation of secondary structures by sgRNA under native conditions it is necessary to run this gel under denaturing conditions. A representative image for injection ready sgRNA under different concentrations is shown in Fig. 1c (left) and an example for degraded sgRNA is shown in Fig. 1c (right).

1. Clean your entire electrophoresis system (including combs and casting system) with RNase surface decontaminant and subsequently fill it with 1× MOPS running buffer.

2. Make an agarose gel by mixing 0.7 g of RNAse-free agarose with 50 mL of DEPC-treated water. Ensure that you use baked (RNase-free) glassware for preparation of this gel.

3. Boil the mixture by microwaving until agarose is dissolved and the mixture is completely translucent. Let cool down to 60 °C.

4. Add 5.9 mL 10× MOPS and 1.8 mL 37% formaldehyde, pour the gel in the casting system and let solidify.

5. Mix 1 μL of each sgRNA with 4 μL of RNA loading buffer. Mix 2 μL of the RiboRuler High Range RNA Ladder with 8 μL of RNA loading buffer. Mix 1 μL of the RiboRuler High Range RNA Ladder with 9 μL of RNA loading buffer. Incubate in a thermoshaker at 65 °C for 5 min. Put on ice **immediately** after incubation for at least 2 min.

6. Load the gel with the samples and the ladders. Run until separation of the ladder is apparent on the employed electrophoresis system.

7. Visualize the gel by appropriate method. As the GelRed is an in-sample stain, no post-stain is required and visualization can thus be performed immediately after running. Make sure to save this gel image digitally for sgRNA quantification purposes (*see* Subheading 3.2.4).

3.2.4 sgRNA Quantification

Accurate quantification of sgRNAs after in vitro transcription is not at all straightforward. We have tested several methods such as NanoDrop (ThermoFisher Scientific), Qubit BR RNA assay (ThermoFisher Scientific), DropSense (Trinean), and Fragment Analyzer (Advanced Analytical). None of these seemed to accurately reflect (diverging by magnitudes of at least two) the amounts of sgRNA that could be estimated by regression curve comparison using the two dilutions of the quantitative ladder on a denaturing gel electrophoresis (unpublished work). Furthermore, we have observed that the Qubit system underestimates the sgRNA yield at least tenfold, but it does accurately measure the proportional differences in yield between different sgRNA synthesis reactions (*see* **Note 8**). In conclusion, for absolute quantification we thus recommend regression curve based quantification of the sgRNA based on the comparison with known standards on a denaturing gel. For multiplex CRISPR/Cas9 experiments (coinjections of more than one sgRNA), however, an additional concern is to provide equimolar amounts of each sgRNA in the injection mixture, this in order to ensure that not a single sgRNA will be overrepresented and thus predominantly bind the available Cas9 protein during the precomplexing of the mixture prior to microinjection. As such, we employ the Qubit system to accurately ensure a 1:1 molar ratio of each gRNA in the injection mixture, this while we are aware that the exact quantitative output of the Qubit system is not correct.

1. Quantify your sgRNA yield by comparing the intensity of the two dilutions of the RiboRuler High Range RNA Ladder bands of known concentration (see manufacturer's instruction) to the intensity of the sgRNA bands by digital analysis of the denaturing gel image obtained in Subheading 3.2.3. We use regression curve based "absolute quantification" under the "quantity tools" in Image Lab 5.2.1.

2. Quantify your sgRNA yield by Qubit RNA BR Assay Kit according to the manufacturer's instructions.

3.3 Delivery of sgRNA/Cas9 Ribonucleoproteins by Microinjection to Xenopus tropicalis Embryos

Here we discuss delivery of the CRISPR/Cas9 system to the developing *Xenopus tropicalis* embryo. Firstly, we would like to mention that although efficient genome editing has been shown by coinjections of Cas9 mRNA together with sgRNA, we and others have observed a dramatic increase in CRISPR/Cas9 mediated genome editing efficiency when employing recombinant Cas9 protein [18]. The sgRNA is thus delivered together with Cas9 protein as a pre-complexed Cas9/gRNA Ribonucleoprotein (RNP). We also show how to set up your injection mixtures if targeting more than one member of the retinoblastoma family by multiplex CRISPR/Cas9 technology.

1. Obtain fertilized *X. tropicalis* embryos, either by natural matings (*see* **Note 9**) or by in vitro fertilization techniques [26, 27].

2. After fertilization, obtain microinjection ready embryos by removing the jelly coat. Discard the buffer containing the embryos and replace with 2% cysteine solution. Swirl the embryos within their recipient to ensure equal exposure to the cysteine solution. Thoroughly wash (four times) embryos with 0.1× MMR solution.

3. Generate the injection mix by combining sgRNA and Cas9 protein to obtain a final concentration of 20–1000 ng/μL sgRNA and 500–1000 ng/μL of Cas9 protein. Optimal concentrations are dependent on the specific sgRNA employed. As a good starting point we suggest 100 ng/μL of (each) sgRNA mixed with 800 ng/μL of Cas9 protein. For multiplex CRISPR/Cas9 obtain a dilution factor for one sgRNA from the values obtained from the denaturing gel electrophoresis with standard regression curve based quantification to the desired end concentration. Then employ the ratio between the Qubit quantification for each employed sgRNA to calculate the desired dilution factor for the other sgRNAs in the mix, thus ensuring a 1:1 molar ratio of the gRNAs (*see* **Note 10** for an example calculation).

4. Incubate the injection mixture at 37 °C for 1 min immediately before loading the mixture in the microinjection needle. This allows preformation of the sgRNA/Cas9 ribonucleoprotein complex and maximization of mutagenesis as described by Burger et al. [28].

5. Place embryos in 6% Ficoll/0.1× MMR solution during the microinjection procedure.

6. Deliver by microinjection 1 nL of injection mix in one blastomere of the two-cell stage *X. tropicalis* embryo, thus delivering 20–1000 pg of each gRNA with 500–1000 pg of Cas9 (w/NLS) protein.

7. Both injected and noninjected embryos should be kept overnight in 6% Ficoll/0.1× MMR.

8. The next day, carefully wash (3×) surviving embryos with 0.1× MMR and remove any dead embryos. *X. tropicalis* should be raised further as described before by Tran Thi et al. [29].

3.4 Assessment of Genome Editing in F0 Mosaic Mutant X. tropicalis

Several tools have been described for assessing genome editing efficiency such as surveyor assay [30], T7 endonuclease I (T7E1) [31], fragment analysis [18], high resolution melting curve analysis (HRMA) and heteroduplex mobility assay (HMA) [32]. We employ HMA as a rapid and cost-effective qualitative method of initial genome modification assessment. However, HMA is not quantitative while surveyor assay, T7E1 and fragment analysis allow for crude estimations of genome editing efficiencies. Nevertheless, HMA has distinct advantages as it allows for detection of very small genome editing efficiencies (below 2%) while for surveyor assay, T7E1 and HRMA, respectively, detection limits of 5%, 20% and 4.7% have been reported [33–35]. For assessment of genome editing when targeting tumor suppressors, the HMA method is thus highly relevant as the positive selection system that is tumorigenesis does not require high mutations efficiencies and additionally high efficiencies might be deleterious to normal embryonal development [36, 37]. Recently, it has been shown by Boel et al. that batch analysis of next-generation sequencing data (BATCH-GE) can provide a rapid and very cost-effective platform for quantitative evaluation of CRISPR/Cas9 based experiments [38]. We now routinely use next-generation sequencing and BATCH-GE analysis to obtain accurate quantification of genome editing efficiencies and specific frequencies of each sequence variant within the complete mosaic F0 animal or within specific dissected tissues.

3.4.1 Obtaining Genomic DNA by Lysis

Embryos can be lysed as early as 24 h post-injection (*see* **Note 11**). Technically, tadpoles can be lysed at any stage to assess genome editing efficiencies, but practical constraints (size, yolk) culminate in optimal lysis around stage 33–36. In order to average out the possible fluctuations in editing efficiency between different tadpoles within the same setup, we pool five to ten embryos and perform the genotyping on these pools.

1. Transfer injected and WT embryos to 100 μL lysis buffer.

2. Lyse overnight at 55 °C on a thermoshaker.

3. Heat for 5 min at 99 °C to inactivate proteinase K.

4. Spin down at 14,000 RPM for 1 min on a standard bench-top centrifuge.

Heteroduplex mobility assay (HMA) is based on the phenomenon that the cells of the mosaic mutant F0 animal will exhibit either wild type (WT) or small insertion-deletion (INDEL) variants, on one or both of the targeted alleles. After amplifying the CRISPR/Cas9 targeted site by PCR, the solution is heated to denature the PCR products and subsequently a slow cooling is performed to allow DNA fragments to anneal even if they are not completely complementary thus forming heteroduplex DNA in addition to homoduplex DNA [32]. This mixture is separated on a polyacrylamide gel electrophoresis system. Heteroduplex bands can be detected in correctly gene-edited samples when compared to WT samples due their specific differential migration patterns. As such, HMA is a fast and short hands-on time method for qualitative assessment of genome editing [34].

1. Design primers to amplify a region of 300–500 bp around the sgRNA cut site (*see* **Note 12** for upper and lower limits of primer design).

2. Test these primers by performing a standard proof-reading PCR on WT DNA and separate the resulting product by 1% agarose gel electrophoresis. Confirm presence of on-target fragment and absence of any off-target fragments. This step is quintessential as aspecific products can interfere with correct interpretation of your HMA gel and can render a false negative result.

3. Perform HMA PCR on WT DNA and DNA from injected tadpoles. We recommend taking at least two samples for each setup as this simplifies interpretation of the resulting data. Run following PCR program with a proof-reading polymerase (such as Phusion polymerase) in a thermocycler: 98 °C for 3 min; 35 cycles of [98 °C for 30 s; x °C for 30 s; 72 °C for 15 s]; 72 °C for 4 min; 98 °C for 5 min, controlled cool-down to 4 °C at a ramp rate of 1 °C/sec]. The annealing temperature x is evidently dependent on the designed primer pair.

4. Cast TBE-buffered acrylamide gel on your polyacrylamide gel electrophoresis apparatus in following proportions:

1× TBE buffer	12 mL
40% Acrylamide–Bis-acrylamide	3 mL
10% APS	140 μL
TEMED	14 μL

5. Mix the PCR products with DNA loading dye and load these on gel. Take care to load the PCR products from the noninjected samples immediately adjacent to the products from the injected samples.

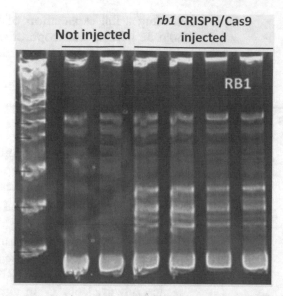

Fig. 2 Heteroduplex Mobility Assay (HMA) demonstrates in a qualitative manner genome editing by *rb1* CRISPR/Cas9. When comparing the "not injected" and "*rb1* CRISPR/Cas9 injected" samples, it is clear that the *rb1* target site has been edited by the CRISPR/Cas9 system which leads in this assay to the detection of extra heteroduplex bands. The employed ladder is the BenchTop 1 kb DNA Ladder (Promega)

6. Run the TBE-buffered polyacrylamide gel for 3–4 h at 50–60 V.

7. Post-stain the gel with GelRed at working stock diluted in purified water and visualize by appropriate methods.

8. If CRISPR/Cas9 genome editing was successful one should clearly observe the presence of additional bands in the injected samples when compared to the noninjected samples. These heteroduplex bands are indicative of effective genome editing. A representative gel image for a qualitative check of genome editing at the *rb1* locus is shown in Fig. 2.

3.4.3 Quantitative Assessment of Genome Editing Efficiencies by Targeted Deep Sequencing and BATCH-GE Analysis

We employ next-generation sequencing in order to obtain a quantitative assessment of genome editing. For this we employ the same primers as have been used for the HMA analysis (*see* Subheading 3.4.2). The specific amplified fragment is subsequently shipped out for MiSeq next-generation sequencing. All following steps are not performed in-house and are thus outsourced to a sequencing facility. Nevertheless, in short, the BATCH-GE method consists out of raw equimolar pooling and library preparation of singleplex PCRs, which are subsequently sequenced by illumina sequencing. Implementation of the BATCH-GE algorithm on the resulting raw data allows accurate detection of genome editing efficiencies and frequencies of each specific mutation within the sequenced pool.

Providing a full explanation of how to implement this protocol would be beyond the scope of this chapter, but we would like to point readers interested in setting up this system to the recent paper by Boel et al. [38].

4   Notes

1. Velocity HiFi polymerase and the corresponding reaction buffer can be replaced by another proofreading and low error polymerase. The DNA template synthesis reaction works equally well by exchanging the Velocity in this reaction by Phusion polymerase.

2. We have only had experience in our hands by side-by-side comparison sgRNA of these two kits. Both performed well for in vitro transcription of sgRNAs. Please note that not all commercially available T7 in vitro transcription kits are amenable to generate RNA as small as sgRNAs are. As such we cannot vouch for the efficiency for sgRNA synthesis efficiencies using any other kits than the ones we mentioned before. This being said, some might perform equally well but this is not tested nor known on our behalves.

3. This specific PCR cleanup kit works very well for cleanup of small DNA templates in the context of sgRNA synthesis. We have tested one other kit (Machery-Nagel) that did not yield desirable outcomes. We believe you can attempt using your favorite PCR cleanup kit for this, and it might work well. However, if you observe low or impure yields, use the suggested Purelink kit or perform traditional phenol–chloroform extraction and sodium acetate EtOH precipitation as described in Subheading 3.2.2.

4. As minor traces of DNA template contaminations within the sgRNA/Cas9 injection mixture can potentially lead to embryonal toxicity we employ TURBO™ DNase, this considering it is more efficient at removing DNA template when compared to traditional DNase I (see manufacturer's instructions).

5. We have performed extensive side-by-side comparisons of several staining methods on denaturing gels (sgRNA quality control) and HMA polyacrylamide gels (assessment of genome editing). We tested EtBr, SYBR safe, SERVA DNA stain G, SERVA DNA stain Clear G, Gel Red, Gel Green, Midori Green Advance and Midori Green Direct. We have observed that only EtBr and Gel Red render clear and interpretable bands using the methods we provide in this book chapter. Considering the toxic profile of EtBr we recommend employing Gel Red diluted in the NorthernMax® Formaldehyde Load Dye.

6. If possible, use sgRNAs that score higher than 50 in the CRISPRScan algorithm. If you cannot identify high-scoring targets it is, however, still feasible to continue with some lower scoring ones. As this is an in silico prediction, this indicates that the higher the score the higher the expected chance of success defined as a highly effective sgRNA at that site. In line with this, an sgRNA with a lower score might have a reduced chance of success. However, this does not formally imply that it will not work.

7. The CRISPRScan algorithm only outputs oligos with 5'-GG allowing for in vitro transcription. However, if employing a different sgRNA design algorithm make sure to either: (1) select targets starting with 5'-GG, or (2) add GG in front of target sequence (we have experimentally observed that this overhang addition does not interfere with sgRNA target site recognition).

8. We suspect this underestimation to be the consequence of the Qubit fluorescent dyes not binding to the sgRNA target molecules due to the specific inherent secondary structures of the sgRNA molecule. As such, the measurement will highly underestimate the total sgRNA yield. Nevertheless, as the inherent secondary structure formation of the sgRNAs should be more or less identical between different sgRNAs we nevertheless believe this to be a powerful method for determining 1:1 molar ratios for sgRNAs.

9. *X. tropicalis* matings are performed essentially as described by the Grainger lab (http://faculty.virginia.edu/xtropicalis/husbandry/mating.html). However, we employ a reduced amount of HCG for priming and boosting. Priming is performed by administering 10 Units HCG to males and 20 Units HCG to females. Boosting is performed by administering 100 Units HCG to males and 150 Units HCG to females.

10. Case study example: We want to coinject sgRNA x and y and thus want to obtain an injection mix containing 100 ng/μL of each sgRNA at a 1:1 molar ratio. sgRNA x is quantified at 2 μg/μL on denaturing gel and at 170 ng/μL on Qubit. sgRNA y is quantified at 2.5 μg/μL on denaturing gel and at 240 ng/μL on Qubit. We thus employ the denaturing gel quantification to decide on a dilution factor of 20 for sgRNA x in the final injection mixture. Considering the qubit is more accurate at determining 1:1 sgRNA molar ratios we choose not to dilute sgRNA by 25 times, but to dilute it approximately 28 times in the final injection mixture. As such, your injection mixture contains 1:1 amounts according to Qubit (each sgRNA final at 8.5 ng/μL) while we know that these correspond to real life values of around 100 ng/μL according to the denaturing gel quantification.

11. When lysing early stage embryos there will be a visually apparent layer of yolk present on top of the aqueous phase containing your genomic DNA of interest. Beware not to transfer this into downstream reactions (PCRs, etc.) as it will interfere with these. Fast pipetting can ensure clean transfer of lysed aqueous phase and yolk attached on the outside of the pipette tip should be removed by wiping with a Tork paper.

12. When encountering difficulties to design primers for amplification of your CRISPR/Cas9 target sequence it is possible to go as high as an amplicon size of 900 bp. Beware however, that when running your HMA, the homoduplexes and heteroduplexes will need longer to separate and thus respect the rule that: the larger your amplicon, the longer your HMA will have to run in order to give unambiguous data (can be up to 5 h for large amplicons).

Acknowledgments

The authors would like to thank Rivka Noelanders for critical proofreading of the chapter. Thomas Naert holds a PhD fellowship with VLAIO-HERMES. Research in the authors' laboratory is supported by the Research Foundation—Flanders (FWO-Vlaanderen; Grant # G.0D87.16N), by the Belgian Science Policy (Interuniversity Attraction Poles—IAP7/07) and by the Desmoid Tumor Research Foundation. Further support was obtained by the Hercules Foundation, Flanders (grant AUGE/11/14) and Concerted Research Actions from Ghent University (BOF15/GOA/011).

References

1. Abramson DH (2005) Retinoblastoma in the 20th century: past success and future challenges the Weisenfeld lecture. Invest Ophthalmol Vis Sci 46:2683–2691

2. Knudson AG Jr (1971) Mutation and cancer: statistical study of retinoblastoma. Proc Natl Acad Sci U S A 68:820–823

3. Cavenee WK et al (1983) Expression of recessive alleles by chromosomal mechanisms in retinoblastoma. Nature 305:779–784

4. Friend SH et al (1986) A human DNA segment with properties of the gene that predisposes to retinoblastoma and osteosarcoma. Nature 323:643–646

5. Stratton MR et al (1989) Structural alterations of the *RB1* gene in human soft tissue tumours. Br J Cancer 60:202–205

6. Harbour JW et al (1988) Abnormalities in structure and expression of the human retinoblastoma gene in SCLC. Science 241:353–357

7. Creytens D et al (2014) Atypical spindle cell lipoma: a clinicopathologic, immunohistochemical, and molecular study emphasizing its relationship to classical spindle cell lipoma. Virchows Arch 465:97–108

8. Pleasance ED et al (2010) A small-cell lung cancer genome with complex signatures of tobacco exposure. Nature 463:184–190

9. Jakobiec FA, Tso MO, Zimmerman LE, Danis P (1977) Retinoblastoma and intracranial malignancy. Cancer 39:2048–2058

10. Marcus DM et al (1998) Trilateral retinoblastoma: insights into histogenesis and management. Surv Ophthalmol 43:59–70

11. MacPherson D et al (2004) Cell type-specific effects of Rb deletion in the murine retina. Genes Dev 18:1681–1694

12. Zhang J, Schweers B, Dyer MA (2004) The first knockout mouse model of retinoblastoma. Cell Cycle 3:952–959

13. Chen D et al (2004) Cell-specific effects of RB or RB/p107 loss on retinal development implicate an intrinsically death-resistant cell-of-origin in retinoblastoma. Cancer Cell 5:539–551

14. Xie C et al (2015) Co-deleting Pten with Rb in retinal progenitor cells in mice results in fully penetrant bilateral retinoblastomas. Mol Cancer 14:93

15. Nakayama T et al (2014) Cas9-based genome editing in Xenopus tropicalis. Methods Enzymol 546:355–375

16. Abu-Daya A, Khokha MK, Zimmerman LB (2012) The hitchhiker's guide to Xenopus genetics. Genesis 50:164–175

17. Naert T, van Nieuwenhuysen T, Vleminckx K (2017) TALENs and CRISPR/Cas9 fuel genetically engineered clinically relevant Xenopus tropicalis tumor models. Genesis 55:e23005

18. Bhattacharya D, Marfo CA, Li D, Lane M, Khokha MK (2015) CRISPR/Cas9: an inexpensive, efficient loss of function tool to screen human disease genes in Xenopus. Dev Biol 408:196–204

19. Van Nieuwenhuysen T et al (2015) TALEN-mediated apc mutation in *Xenopus tropicalis* phenocopies familial adenomatous polyposis. Oncoscience 2:555–566

20. Naert T et al (2016) CRISP/Cas9 mediated knockout of rb1 and rbl1 leads to rapid and penetrant retinoblastoma development in *Xenopus tropicalis*. Sci Rep 6:35263

21. Stemmer M, Thumberger T, Del Sol Keyer M, Wittbrodt J, Mateo JL (2015) CCTop: an intuitive, flexible and reliable CRISPR/Cas9 target prediction tool. PLoS One 10:e0124633

22. Doench JG et al (2014) Rational design of highly active sgRNAs for CRISPR-Cas9-mediated gene inactivation. Nat Biotechnol 32:1262–1267

23. Moreno-Mateos MA et al (2015) CRISPRscan: designing highly efficient sgRNAs for CRISPR-Cas9 targeting in vivo. Nat Methods 12:982–988

24. Popp MW, Maquat LE (2016) Leveraging rules of nonsense-mediated mRNA decay for genome engineering and personalized medicine. Cell 165:1319–1322

25. Cobrinik D (2005) Pocket proteins and cell cycle control. Oncogene 24:2796–2809

26. Showell C, Conlon FL (2009) Natural mating and tadpole husbandry in the western clawed frog *Xenopus tropicalis*. Cold Spring Harb Protoc 2009:pdb prot5292

27. Showell C, Conlon FL (2009) Egg collection and *in vitro* fertilization of the western clawed frog *Xenopus tropicalis*. Cold Spring Harb Protoc 2009:pdb prot5293

28. Burger A et al (2016) Maximizing mutagenesis with solubilized CRISPR-Cas9 ribonucleoprotein complexes. Development 143:2025–2037

29. Tran HT, Vleminckx K (2014) Design and use of transgenic reporter strains for detecting activity of signaling pathways in Xenopus. Methods 66:422–432

30. Qiu P et al (2004) Mutation detection using Surveyor nuclease. Biotechniques 36:702–707

31. Babon JJ, McKenzie M, Cotton RG (2003) The use of resolvases T4 endonuclease VII and T7 endonuclease I in mutation detection. Mol Biotechnol 23:73–81

32. Upchurch DA, Shankarappa R, Mullins JI (2000) Position and degree of mismatches and the mobility of DNA heteroduplexes. Nucleic Acids Res 28:E69

33. Vouillot L, Thelie A, Pollet N (2015) Comparison of T7E1 and surveyor mismatch cleavage assays to detect mutations triggered by engineered nucleases. G3 (Bethesda) 5:407–415

34. Zhu X et al (2014) An efficient genotyping method for genome-modified animals and human cells generated with CRISPR/Cas9 system. Sci Rep 4:6420

35. Thomas HR, Percival SM, Yoder BK, Parant JM (2014) High-throughput genome editing and phenotyping facilitated by high resolution melting curve analysis. PLoS One 9:e114632

36. Clarke AR et al (1992) Requirement for a functional Rb-1 gene in murine development. Nature 359:328–330

37. Lee EY et al (1992) Mice deficient for Rb are nonviable and show defects in neurogenesis and haematopoiesis. Nature 359:288–294

38. Boel A et al (2016) BATCH-GE: batch analysis of next-generation sequencing data for genome editing assessment. Sci Rep 6:30330

INDEX

Pedro G. Santiago-Cardona (ed.), *The Retinoblastoma Protein*, Methods in Molecular Biology, vol. 1726,
https://doi.org/10.1007/978-1-4939-7565-5, © Springer Science+Business Media, LLC 2018